Essentials of Dementia

Essentials of Dementia

Everything You Really Need to Know for Working in Dementia Care

Dr Shibley Rahman and **Professor Rob Howard**

Forewords by **Karen Harrison Dening and Kate Swaffer**

Jessica Kingsley *Publishers*
London and Philadelphia

Disclaimer: Every effort has been made to ensure that the information contained in this book is correct, but it should not in any way be substituted for medical, regulatory or legal advice. Readers should always consult a qualified medical practitioner before adopting any complementary or alternative therapies. Neither the author nor the publisher takes responsibility for any consequences of any decision made as a result of the information contained in this book.

First published in 2018
by Jessica Kingsley Publishers
73 Collier Street
London N1 9BE, UK
and
400 Market Street, Suite 400
Philadelphia, PA 19106, USA

www.jkp.com

Copyright © Dr Shibley Rahman and Professor Rob Howard 2018
Foreword copyright © Karen Harrison Dening 2018
Foreword copyright © Kate Swaffer 2018

Library of Congress Cataloging in Publication Data
A CIP catalog record for this book is available from the Library of Congress

British Library Cataloguing in Publication Data
A CIP catalogue record for this book is available from the British Library

ISBN 978 1 78592 397 5
eISBN 978 1 78450 754 1

Printed and bound in the United States

Contents

Foreword

Karen Harrison Dening

It is a pleasure to be asked to write a foreword for this book. I have worked in the field of dementia care for much longer than I care to admit but, if I had access to literature of this quality as I set out on my career in working with families affected by dementia, I would have been well-prepared.

To be able to work competently with families affected by dementia we have needed to move beyond the platitudes of dementia awareness and into the realms of dementia literacy and knowledge. There has been much work and debate on what competency in dementia care looks like; what levels of knowledge might be required by professionals in different settings; tiers and hierarchy in levels of skill and knowledge dependent upon the degree of engagement; and curriculum content for such levels.

A novel approach and a real strength of this book is how its sections specifically relate to individual National Occupational Standards. The National Occupational Standards (NOS) describe best practice across health and social care by bringing together the skills, knowledge and values required, in this instance, to meet the care needs of families affected by dementia.[1] There are over 200 separate NOS that can be grouped to cover all sorts of roles and also different levels of responsibility. This book cleverly cross-matches relevant NOS to enable the reader to further develop their knowledge and skills in order to meet those standards.

Educational texts can often be dry in their presentation but this book has a punchy style that offers bite-sized pieces of information, which makes the information easy to access and relate to practice. Whilst each chapter is a stand-alone treatise on important aspects of dementia care, there are some that resonated with me as the reader. As an example, I particularly like Chapter 2, which discusses dementia and its sub-types. The authors go beyond the broad 'dementia awareness' descriptions of dementia and offer us a little more science into the mix – not too much but just enough. Enough to add interest but not so much it skims over the reader's understanding.

This distinguished pair of authors are to be congratulated in bringing together the 'need to know' elements of the NOS and relating these to the knowledge and information required to enable the health and social care student/practitioner to meet those standards.

This text would be an essential book on the shelf of all health and social care academic departments but, more so, on the bookshelf of each health and social care professional working in the field of dementia care. Oh that it had been available during my own training!

Karen Harrison Dening
Head of Research and Publications, Dementia UK

Notes

1. www.skillsforcare.org.uk/Standards-legislation/National-Occupational-Standards

Foreword

Kate Swaffer

As a retired nurse, past care partner for three people with dementia, and one of eight co-founders of Dementia Alliance International, a 'patient' advocacy and support group, of, by and for people with dementia, it is an honour to introduce this book. The health care sector, including general practitioners, nurses and service providers, are not as well-educated in dementia as other health conditions, for example heart disease or cancer, and this book will help to plug that gap.

The World Health Organization (WHO) provides this definition: 'Dementia is a syndrome in which there is deterioration in memory, thinking, behaviour and the ability to perform everyday activities.'[1] John Sandblom,[2] co-founder of Dementia Alliance International, sees dementia differently: 'We are just changing in ways the rest of you aren't, we have increasing disabilities and the sooner it is looked at that way instead of the stigmas, misunderstandings…the better for all of us living with dementia. We desperately need others to enable us, not further disable us!' I see 'dementia' as 'a group of diseases or conditions, whereby the symptoms must be seen and supported as cognitive disAbilities, and therefore all people with dementia have a human right to proactive disAbility support, including physical and cognitive rehabilitation'. The WHO now also officially recognises them as cognitive disAbilities.

What this book brings to students is a unique and comprehensive medical overview of dementia, and many of the essential care principles. In Chapter 3, when discussing person-centred care, the 'VIPS framework' is also referred to, to assist people in thinking about how to translate person-centred care into practice. I believe all care interventions and strategies need to ensure people with dementia are living positively, either in the community or in residential care.

What I really like is that this book covers topics such as the physical environment, and how important it is for helping people with dementia maintain independence and dignity. The discussion on the cultural appropriateness of care is also quite unique for a medical book of this type, and important for everyone working in this sector. Chapter 5 on communication is also exceptional in this genre of book, as rarely is the importance of communication skills discussed, especially in terms of the cause of changed responses or behaviours.

The book covers the use of pharmacological interventions, including antipsychotics, and makes it very clear that they should be used with great caution, and only under the close and regular supervision of appropriate medical doctors. The book also reviews the many non-pharmacological interventions and approaches to more positively support people with dementia with unmet needs, clarifying that much more research is needed in this field.

It is ahead of its time, as it is well-aligned to a number of the seven cross-cutting principles in the 'Global action plan on the public health response to dementia',[3] which was only adopted in May 2017 at the World Health Assembly. These seven cross-cutting principles include:

1. Human rights of people with dementia

2. Empowerment and engagement of people with dementia and their care partners

3. Evidence-based practice for dementia risk reduction and care

4. Multisector collaboration on the public health response to dementia

5. Universal health and social care coverage for dementia

6. Equity

7. Appropriate attention to dementia prevention, cure and care.

Therefore, it is my hope that those people developing national or regional dementia strategies and plans will also refer to this book. Chapter 8 on living well with dementia is a complementary section supporting the global action plan, and is very relevant to national and regional strategies and plans, and also to the dementia-friendly communities movement.

What makes this book so distinctive compared to other medical dementia books is that it provides teachings that address dementia beyond the medical definition, and education and strategies for us to live with dementia; not only to go home and die from it.

Thank you, Dr Rahman and Professor Howard. As one of the estimated 50 million people globally living with dementia, this is hugely important to me personally, but also to all people with dementia and our families.

Kate Swaffer
Author and Activist; Chair, CEO and Co-founder, Dementia Alliance International; Member, World Dementia Council; Board Member, Alzheimer's Disease International; PhD Candidate, University of Wollongong

Notes

1. www.who.int/mediacentre/factsheets/fs362/en
2. https://www.dementiaallianceinternational.org
3. https://www.alz.co.uk/media/170529

Acknowledgements

Thanks to all people who've read this manuscript. We have tried to include all your suggestions for improvement.

Preface

Education, training and skills acquisition are hallmarks of good dementia care.

Dementia represents one of the biggest global health problems facing society today. Proposed dementia care pathways involve many disciplines and health sectors, and a global priority is the continuing education of professionals delivering care.[1] In other words, 'dementia awareness' should definitely apply to all practitioners and professionals too.

The aim is to support all professionals and practitioners to be responsive to the needs of people with dementia, to continue to develop their skills and expertise, and to improve the contribution they make to achieving the best outcomes for people with dementia, their care partners and families.

In England, it is estimated that around 676,000 people have dementia. In the whole of the UK, the number of people with dementia is 850,000.[2]

At the heart of the challenge is a workforce not properly equipped to work with people with dementia. Key stakeholders are, however, beginning to respond to the agenda.

Some time ago, the Alzheimer's Society[3] found that people with dementia were staying in hospital longer than those without dementia, with a detrimental impact on the individual's dementia and physical health. Around the same time, the Department of Health published 'Living well with dementia: A National Dementia Strategy' for England, which committed to developing an informed and effective workforce as a key element in delivering the strategy.[4]

It is widely believed that to support people in living well with dementia, we need to continue to make progress on improving awareness and understanding of the condition to transform the way society thinks and acts about dementia. Every organisation and every person who makes up a community has both a role and a responsibility to act to achieve this.

There is substantial interest from all parts of the health and care spectrum, with a real demand for knowledge, guidelines and information: from prevention to end-of-life care and everything in between.

Dementia Core Skills Education and Training Framework

The Dementia Core Skills Education and Training Framework is an extraordinarily useful resource which details the essential skills and knowledge necessary across the health and social care spectrum.[5]

The Dementia Core Skills Education and Training Framework was commissioned and funded by the Department of Health and developed in collaboration with Skills for Health, Health Education England, Skills for Care and an expert advisory group that ensured multi-organisational and multi-stakeholder representation. Launched in October 2015, it is a comprehensive resource which details the essential skills and knowledge necessary for staff across the broad and varied spectrum of health and social care settings and will support organisations to:

- standardise the interpretation of dementia education and training

- guide the focus and aims of dementia education and training delivery through key learning outcomes

- ensure the educational relevance of dementia training

- improve the quality and consistency of education and training provision.

It sets out standards needed in dementia education and training, including raising dementia awareness, knowledge and skills for those who have regular contact with people affected by dementia, and knowledge and skills for those in leadership roles.

Awareness and 'social action'

Progress has been made on encouraging businesses, local authorities, the wider public sector and civil society to work together to tackle discrimination through their involvement in dementia-friendly communities.

Awareness and social action has already been a phenomenal success with more than two million people becoming 'Dementia Friends', a programme from the Alzheimer's Society (and Public Health England).[6] Dementia awareness and understanding has continued to increase through the creation of an additional 400,000 Dementia Friends and through the launch of Black and Minority Ethnic materials for Dementia Friends.

The five key messages of the successful 'Dementia Friends' programme are:

1. Dementia is not a natural part of ageing.

2. Dementia is caused by diseases of the brain.

3. Dementia is not just about losing your memory.

4. People can continue to live well with dementia.

5. There's always more to the person than his or her dementia.

People aged over 65 now account for over two-thirds of patients in acute hospitals and an increasing number of them will have dementia.[7] Many may be diagnosed with dementia for the first time when admitted to hospital for another reason. As such, all hospitals and physicians who work in them need to be ready to manage all aspects of the care of patients with dementia.

All staff involved in dementia care need to be informed, skilled and have enough time to care. They need to be fully involved in the 'social action' for change. For example:

- All nurses and healthcare assistants need good-quality training and education in dementia that is easy to access, practical and focuses on attitudes, approach and communication with people with dementia.

- Speech and language therapy services should provide equal access to interventions for communication and swallowing disorders. Early speech and language therapy intervention is crucial so that people with dementia and their care partners have their needs met in a timely way.

- Social work is at the heart of empowering people with positive risk-taking approaches and making sure their rights are respected and supported.[8] Social workers seek to build meaningful relationships with people with dementia and their family care partners, making sure they remain at the heart of the decision-making process.

- Occupational therapists evaluate persons with dementia to determine their strengths, impairments and performance areas needing intervention.[9]

- Likewise, physiotherapists can assess problems that restrict a person's physical activities and identify ways in which they can join in with everyday life. They can work with the person with dementia and their care partners to encourage and promote physical activity and maintain their mobility and independence for as long as possible.

Dementia awareness and risk reduction

To date, there has been limited research concerning public perceptions of brain health and how this might affect dementia risk reduction. For example, a national survey undertaken in Australia in 2005 found that popular beliefs about dementia risk were weakly aligned with the scientific evidence, with a low level of understanding about the association between dementia and cardiovascular factors.[10] In addition, even if such links are made, such behaviour change is not always easy.[11]

Raising public awareness of how healthy lifestyle choices can reduce personal risk of developing dementia is a priority. The 'NHS Health Check' includes a mandatory component for raising awareness of dementia for people over the age of 65. But merely providing information about the latest research via educational sessions to health professionals caring for people with dementia may be insufficient to drive change.[12]

New exciting developments

Commissioners in both health and social care need support to improve their awareness of effective practice in the provision of post-diagnostic care and support.

Individuals with dementia who may lack the mental capacity to make their own decisions have their rights enshrined in the Mental Capacity Act 2005 (MCA). Implemented in 2007, the MCA provides opportunities for assisting with planning and making decisions on others' behalf, and may be expected to be entrenched within clinical practice.

Jill Manthorpe and colleagues conducted follow-up qualitative interviews with 15 community-based dementia nurses to detect changes and developments in views and practices of the MCA.[13] It was striking that some participants were concerned about lack of understanding among other professionals and felt more public awareness was required. All providers of care need to be encouraged to make suitable training materials available to their staff.

The World Dementia Council has been re-formed, with a new Chair and Vice Chair, a refreshed membership and terms of reference, and a new, more action-focused operating model. Their aim is to improve awareness of dementia, tackle further risk reduction and prevention, and mitigate against stigma and prejudice.[14]

About this book

You should not take this book to be professional advice. You are also strongly encouraged to read around these subjects in detail to enable you to form your own judgements.

For high-quality dementia care to be provided, we need a workforce that is not only knowledgeable about dementia but also skilled in the provision of care and appreciative of its importance. It is striking that jurisdictions other than the UK have also experienced difficulties in effectively educating their workforce about dementia.

We hope that, whatever your personal and professional background, however little or much you know about dementia, you will find this book informative, interesting and relevant to your needs.

Please let us know what you think of our book, or how you get on with it.

Dr Shibley Rahman (Twitter @dr_shibley)
Prof. Rob Howard (Twitter @profrobhoward)
London, September 2017

Notes

1. World Health Organization (2012) *Dementia: A Public Health Priority.* Geneva, Switzerland: WHO Press. Accessed on 31 August 2017 at www.who.int/mental_health/publications/dementia_report_2012/en
2. NHS England. 'Dementia.' Available at https://www.england.nhs.uk/mental-health/dementia
3. Alzheimer's Society (2009) *Counting the Cost: Caring for People with Dementia on Hospital Wards.* London: Alzheimer's Society. Accessed on 31 August 2017 at www.alzheimers.org.uk/download/downloads/id/787/counting_the_cost.pdf
4. Department of Health (2009) 'Living well with dementia: A National Dementia Strategy.' Accessed on 31 August 2017 at www.gov.uk/government/publications/living-well-with-dementia-a-national-dementia-strategy
5. Dementia Core Skills Education and Training Framework. Accessed on 2 October 2017 at www.skillsforhealth.org.uk/services/item/176-dementia-core-skills-education-and-training-framework
6. Dementia Friends: www.dementiafriends.org.uk.
7. 'Hospitals on the edge? The time for action.' A report by the Royal College of Physicians, September 2012. Accessed on 7 October 2017 at www.rcplondon.ac.uk/guidelines-policy/hospitals-edge-time-action
8. Department of Health (2014) 'A manual for good social work practice: Supporting adults who have dementia.' Accessed on 31 August 2017 at www.gov.uk/government/publications/learning-resource-for-social-work-with-adults-who-have-dementia
9. See, for example, Schaber, P. and Lieberman, D. (2010) *Occupational Therapy Practice Guidelines for Adults with Alzheimer's Disease and Related Disorders.* Bethesda, MD: AOTA Press.
10. Smith, B.J., Ali, S. and Quach, H. (2015) 'The motivation and actions of Australians concerning brain health and dementia risk reduction.' *Health Promotion Journal of Australia 26,* 2, 115–121.
11. O'Donnell, C.A., Browne, S., Pierce, M., McConnachie, A. *et al.* (2015) 'Reducing dementia risk by targeting modifiable risk factors in mid-life: Study protocol for the Innovative Midlife Intervention for Dementia Deterrence (In-MINDD) randomised controlled feasibility trial.' *Pilot and Feasibility Studies 1,* 40, http://doi.org/10.1186/s40814-015-0035-x
12. Goodenough, B., Fleming, R., Young, M., Burns, K., Jones, C. and Forbes, F. (2016) 'Raising awareness of research evidence among health professionals delivering dementia care: Are knowledge translation workshops useful?' *Gerontology and Geriatrics Education 38,* 4, 392–406.
13. Manthorpe, J., Samsi, K. and Rapaport, J. (2014) 'Dementia nurses' experience of the Mental Capacity Act 2005: A follow-up study.' *Dementia (London) 13,* 1, 131–143.
14. World Dementia Council (2017) '*Our Vision and* Mission.' Accessed on 31 August 2017 at https://worlddementiacouncil.org/our-work/our-vision-and-mission

1

Dementia awareness

There were an estimated 46.8 million people worldwide living with dementia in 2015 and this number was believed to be close to 50 million people in 2017.[1]

Dementia is characterised by a complex interaction of cognitive, functional, behavioural and psychological symptoms that decrease the quality of life for both the patient and the care partner.

High-quality informed awareness is crucial – both for members of the public and for practitioners and professionals. Hospitalised people with dementia typically have more advanced disease than those in the community.

However, a recent realist review suggests that strategies such as dementia awareness training alone will not improve dementia care or outcomes for patients with dementia. Instead, how staff are supported to implement learning and resources by senior team members with dementia expertise is a key component for improving care practices and patient outcomes.[2]

It has, for some reason, become very popular to picture dementia as an 'umbrella'.

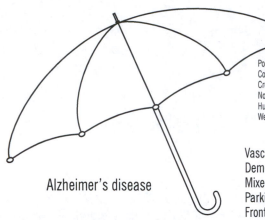

Posterior cortical atrophy
Corticobasal degeneration
Creutzfeldt–Jakob disease and variant
Normal pressure hydrocephalus
Huntington's disease
Wernicke–Korsakoff syndrome

Vascular cognitive impairment
Dementia with Lewy bodies
Mixed dementia
Parkinson's disease dementia
Frontotemporal dementia

Alzheimer's disease

Figure 1.1 Dementia umbrella

What is dementia?

'Dementia' is a word used to describe a group of symptoms that occur when brain cells stop working or die. It is defined as an acquired and progressive loss of a range of cognitive functions that is sufficient to interfere significantly with day-to-day functioning. It's a word that covers more than a hundred different conditions, some of which are very rare and some, like Alzheimer's disease (AD), are very, very common. It is possible to have more than one type of dementia at the same time. Alzheimer's disease is sometimes seen in combination with vascular dementia or dementia with Lewy bodies. You might hear this called 'mixed dementia'.

After Alzheimer's disease, the most common causes of dementia are vascular dementia, dementia with Lewy bodies and frontotemporal dementia. Rarer causes of dementia include posterior cortical atrophy, Wernicke–Korsakoff syndrome, Creutzfeldt–Jakob Disease (CJD) and HIV/AIDS.

Dementia usually develops insidiously and is not always obvious in the early stages. However, some dementias progress very fast.

Dementia is not simply just about memory symptoms. Dementia involves a range of areas of cognition in addition to memory.

If problems are because of dementia, getting a diagnosis has many benefits.

An excellent guide to dementia has been produced by the Alzheimer's Society.[3]

The prevalence of dementia

An important report provided an update of the figures presented in the first edition of *Dementia UK*.[4] It was researched and written by academics from King's College London and the London School of Economics in summer 2014.[5] The key findings were:

- The total age-standardised 65+ population prevalence of dementia was 7.1 per cent (based on population data).

- Using this estimated rate of prevalence, there will have been 850,000 people with dementia in the UK in 2015.

- The total number of people with dementia in the UK is forecast to increase to over one million by 2025 and over two million by 2051 if age-specific prevalence remains stable, and increases are driven by demographic ageing alone.

This provides one important reason why it's important to be aware of dementia as a professional or practitioner. Quite simply, there's a lot of it about.

Signs of dementia

Every person is unique and dementia affects people differently – no two people will have symptoms that appear and develop in exactly the same way. An individual's personality, general health and social situation are all important factors in determining the impact of dementia on him or her and how this will be expressed.

Symptoms vary between Alzheimer's disease and other types of dementia, but there are some similarities between them all.

A person with dementia will have cognitive symptoms (to do with thinking or memory). They will often have problems in some of the following areas:

- **day-to-day memory** – for example, difficulty recalling events or conversations that happened recently

- **concentrating, planning or organising** – for example, difficulties making decisions, solving problems or carrying out a sequence of tasks (such as cooking a meal or dressing)

- **language** – for example, being less fluent, difficulties following a conversation or finding the right word for something

- **visuospatial skills** – for example, problems judging depth or distances (such as on steps and stairs) and seeing patterns or objects in three dimensions – including articles of clothing

- **orientation** – for example, losing track of the day, month or even year, or becoming confused about where they are.

A person with dementia might also have changes in their mood and feelings. For example, they may become frustrated or irritable, apathetic or withdrawn, anxious, easily upset or unusually sad. With some types of dementia, the person may see things that are not really there (visual hallucinations) or strongly believe things that are not true (delusions).

Or it could be that persons with dementia have little insight into their own symptoms, and yet people closest to them notice a definite change in personality and behaviour. And sometimes cognitive thinking – including memory – can appear relatively intact.

Dementia is progressive, which means the symptoms gradually get worse over time. How quickly this happens varies greatly from person to person.

As dementia progresses, the person may develop behaviours that seem unusual or out of character. These behaviours may include asking the same question over and over, pacing, restlessness or agitation and even uncharacteristic aggression. They can be distressing or challenging for the person and very difficult for those close to them.

Dementia can follow 'stages' and one can sometimes talk about the severity of dementia, a reflection of how much function and ability has been affected by the pathology of the dementia. But it would be quite wrong to expect a linear or completely predictable progression of symptoms in any one individual. The 'life course' can vary, reflecting the complexity of genetics as well as the social determinants of health.

In Box 1.1 there is a broad list of symptoms for four very common subtypes of dementia.

BOX 1.1 FEATURES OF THE COMMON DEMENTIAS

Alzheimer's disease

Typical symptoms of early Alzheimer's include:

- regularly forgetting recent events, names and faces
- becoming increasingly repetitive (e.g. repeating questions after a very short interval)
- confusion about the date or time of day
- disorientation, especially away from normal surroundings
- problems finding the right words
- mood or behaviour problems such as apathy, irritability or losing confidence.

Vascular dementia

The early symptoms may be similar to those of Alzheimer's disease. But vascular dementia can have many different symptoms, depending on which area of the brain is affected.

The first symptoms of vascular dementia usually appear gradually but can develop suddenly, depending on the cause. Symptoms of vascular dementia can include:

- memory problems
- disorientation and problems concentrating
- communication problems
- becoming slower in thinking
- changes in mood, behaviour or personality.

Dementia with Lewy bodies

Dementia with Lewy bodies (also known as DLB or Lewy body disease) may affect as many as 125,000 people in the UK.[6]

Symptoms of dementia with Lewy bodies can include:

- fluctuations in attention, alertness and confusion – these fluctuations can be very noticeable from day to day or even hour to hour
- Parkinson's disease-type features, such as slowing or difficulty with walking, hunched posture, stiffness in the limbs and sometimes tremor
- fainting and falls
- delusions
- visual hallucinations and illusions – these can often involve seeing people or animals that aren't really there or misinterpreting patterns or shadows so that illusory faces or objects are seen

- movements during sleep and vivid dreams
- some symptoms similar to Alzheimer's disease, including memory loss and disorientation.

Frontotemporal dementia

Frontotemporal dementia (FTD) describes a number of different conditions. These include behavioural variant FTD, progressive non-fluent aphasia and semantic dementia. FTD is quite rare and tends to have onset in people aged between 45 and 60.

Symptoms of FTD can include:

- personality changes – these may include a change in how people express their feelings towards others or a lack of understanding of other people's feelings
- lack of personal awareness or insight
- changes in social behaviour
- over-eating or changes in dietary preferences (e.g. liking sweet foods and drinks)
- behaviour changes, including developing unusual beliefs, obsessions or compulsions
- difficulty with simple plans and decisions
- decline in language abilities – this might include difficulty understanding words, repeating commonly used words and phrases or forgetting the meaning of words.

Dementia will usually be diagnosed by a specialist doctor such as:

- **a psychiatrist** – a mental health specialist
- **a geriatrician** – a doctor specialising in the health of older people
- **a neurologist** – someone who concentrates on diseases of the nervous system.

Occasionally, a GP or clinical specialist nurse will make the diagnosis, depending on their expertise and training.

There is no single 'test for dementia'. A diagnosis is usually based on a combination of things:

- **taking a 'history'** – the doctor talking to the person and (very importantly) someone who knows them well about how their problems have developed and how they are now affecting their daily life

- **physical examination and tests** (e.g. blood tests) – to exclude other possible causes of the person's symptoms

- **tests of cognitive neuropsychological function** (e.g. memory, thinking, higher-order perception) – simpler tests will be carried out by a nurse or doctor, more specialist tests by a psychologist

- **a scan of the brain** – if this is needed or helpful to make the diagnosis.

A common pattern is for the GP to make an initial assessment and then refer the person to a memory clinic or other specialist service for a more detailed assessment. A specialist doctor will have more expertise in dementia and will be able to arrange more detailed tests and brain scans, if needed.

The diagnosis should be communicated clearly to the person and usually those closest to them as well. There should also be a discussion about the next steps.

Actions individuals can take to reduce their risk of Alzheimer's disease or delay onset

It is unclear whether intellectual, social and physical activities can genuinely improve cognitive performance and protect against dementia, or whether individuals with high-functioning brains are more likely to perform well intellectually and are also protected against the onset of dementia by virtue of their 'cognitive reserve'.

A higher level of education has been traditionally regarded as being protective against age-related cognitive decline and dementia via mechanisms of cognitive reserve. Paradoxically, studies have found a faster rate of decline in Alzheimer's disease patients with higher levels of education. While cognitive reserve may have a protective effect against early presentation of symptoms, this may be lost once the condition has advanced, because higher levels of cognitive reserve may have masked the consequences of large amounts of dementia pathology.

A factor that seems to clearly increase the rate of disease progression is a family history of Alzheimer's disease. Sporadic Alzheimer's disease is distinguished from familial Alzheimer's disease which has known genetic causes. However, appreciation of genetic links to sporadic Alzheimer's disease is increasing. Having an affected first-degree relative with sporadic Alzheimer's disease approximately doubles the risk of developing the condition.

Several studies have examined rigorously the relationship between elevated blood pressure in midlife (age 40–64 years) and the onset of dementia and Alzheimer's disease later in life. Hypertension in midlife is particularly associated with an increased risk of developing dementia. One might hope the treatment of high blood pressure in midlife would reduce the risk of developing dementia, as it does the risk of stroke. It is, however, perhaps less clear how hypertension in later life affects the development of dementia.[7]

Diet is likely to have a 'double-edged sword' effect upon the development and progression of Alzheimer's disease. Diets high in trans-saturated fats and processed sugar and low in polyunsaturated fats and other essential nutrients may contribute to ill health by affecting multiple systems and end-organs; obesity in midlife, for instance, has been identified as a risk factor for Alzheimer's disease. A balanced diet, however, with appropriate levels of vitamins, proteins, polyunsaturated fats and fibre may contribute to healthy ageing.

The Mediterranean diet (MeDi) has been associated with a decrease in the risk of developing Alzheimer's disease. The MeDi is characterised by low levels of saturated fatty acids and sugar, and moderate levels of mono- and polyunsaturated fatty acids from oils, vegetables and fish.

Actions that people affected by dementia can take in order to live as well as possible after diagnosis

There is a wide variety of help and information that should be made available both to people with dementia and to their friends, relatives and care partners.

This dementia support typically includes:

- information on help available at home or in the community, such as from social services, day centres and respite care, community mental health teams, speech and language therapists, dietitians and occupational therapists

- advice regarding financial affairs and planning for the future

- welfare benefits (such as the Personal Independence Payment or Attendance Allowance)

- advice about driving

- advance care planning and help with setting up a lasting power of attorney if the dementia is progressive – this allows a person to be involved in discussions about their future while they are still able to do so effectively

- information and support groups (including local care partners' groups).

The importance of recognising a person with dementia as a unique individual

Someone with dementia, whose mental abilities are declining, will feel vulnerable and in need of reassurance and support. It is important that those around them do everything they can to help them retain their sense of identity and put an emphasis on help with mood and motivation.

Care partners and family should remember that:

- each person with dementia is a unique individual with their own very different experiences of life, their own needs and feelings, and their own likes and dislikes

- each person will be affected by their dementia in a different way

- everyone reacts to the experience of dementia in a different way – the experience means different things to different people.

Those caring for people with dementia will need to take account of the abilities, interests and preferences they have at present, and the fact that these may change as the dementia progresses. They should be prepared to respond in a flexible and sensitive way.

The impact of dementia on individuals, families and society

Nobody should be given a diagnosis of dementia alone – a diagnosis of dementia also affects close friends and family.

Dementia also has a huge impact on society, but the human value of the lives of individuals with dementia is crucial.

A powerful narrative based on citizenship and human rights of people with dementia is crystallising fast. The impact that dementia has on people's ability to participate in daily activities and its relationship to health and wellbeing has tended to be overlooked or underestimated.

Some of the most common feelings families and care partners experience are guilt, grief and loss, and a sense of anger. Patterns of grief are not necessarily easily predictable, and care partners can experience a sense of grief and bereavement even before the death of their loved one.

While grief is a normal experience following a major loss, family care partners' grief can become complicated or prolonged when a person experiences cognitive, behavioural and emotional distress causing impairment in social functioning and performance for some time following a bereavement.

The importance of communicating effectively and compassionately with individuals who have dementia

It's important not to make a person with dementia feel awkward by telling him or her that he or she has 'already said that within the last few minutes', or to question him or her on recent events.

In short, for healthcare professionals, compassion means seeing the *person* in the patient at all times and at all points of care, and to behave with compassion and patience wherever possible.

Why a person with dementia may exhibit signs of distress and how behaviours seen in people with dementia may be a means for communicating unmet needs

A person may exhibit signs of 'distress' through their behaviour, particularly if he or she is having difficulty in expressing himself or herself, verbally or non-verbally.

There are simple things you can do, including asking the person with dementia what the matter is, what he or she is feeling and what he or she ideally would like you to do to help.

People with dementia might say that they withdraw from social activities because of feelings of embarrassment and stress in social situations due to cognitive lapses and difficulty keeping up with conversations and/or activities. Furthermore, social withdrawal can increase if they experience negative reactions from others in social contexts, such as the experiences previously presented and the concept of malignant social psychology, and can serve to reinforce negative self-concepts.

How to signpost individuals, families and care partners to dementia advice, support and information

---

BOX 1.2 NATIONAL OCCUPATIONAL STANDARDS ON SIGNPOSTING

National Occupational Standard SCDHSC0026 – 'Support individuals to access information on services and facilities' – includes supporting the individual to use information you supply, to access and use information themselves and then to evaluate and feed back on it.

National Occupational Standard SCDHSC0419 – 'Provide advice and information to those who enquire about health and social care services' – identifies the requirements when you provide advice and information about health and social care services, including identifying the person's requirements in providing advanced information about health and social care services, ensuring continuous quality improvement in service provision.

Signposting is when a health professional or other expert makes a person with dementia or someone close to them aware of other services, provides information in the form of a leaflet or booklet, or tells the person where they can obtain further information or support. For example, a person may wish to know about a specific psychosocial intervention.

Signposting can include information about useful websites, local groups and courses, social media 'role models', and other support and services available in a local area.

Notes

1.   Alzheimer's Disease International (2015) 'Dementia statistics.' Accessed on 6 November 2017 at www.alz.co.uk/research/statistics
2.   Handley, M., Bunn, F., Goodman, C. (2017) 'Dementia-friendly interventions to improve the care of people living with dementia admitted to hospitals: A realist review.' *BMJ Open 7*, e015257. doi: 10.1136/bmjopen-2016-015257.
3.   Alzheimer's Society (2017) 'The dementia guide: Living well after diagnosis.' Accessed on 31 August 2017 at www.alzheimers.org.uk/download/downloads/id/1881/the_dementia_guide. pdf
4.   Alzheimer's Society (2007) *Dementia UK 2007.* Accessed on 31 August 2017 at www.alzheimers. org.uk/downloads/download/1/dementia_uk_2007

5. Alzheimer's Society (2014) *Dementia UK Update.* Accessed on 7 October at www.alzheimers.org. uk/download/downloads/id/2323/dementia_uk_update.pdf
6. Alzheimer's Research UK. 'All about dementia.' Available at https://www.alzheimersresearchuk. org/wp-content/uploads/2015/01/All-about-dementia.pdf
7. Kennelly, S.P., Lawlor, B.A. and Kenny, R.A. (2009) 'Blood pressure and dementia – a comprehensive review.' *Ther Adv Neurol Disord 2*, 4, 241–260.

2

Dementia identification, assessment and diagnosis

The symptoms of dementia are caused when the brain is damaged by disease. Alzheimer's disease is the most common cause of dementia, but not the only one (see below). The specific symptoms that someone with dementia experiences will depend on the parts of the brain that are damaged and the disease that is causing the dementia.

The most common types of dementia in the UK

Dementia is a syndrome (essentially irreversible and progressive 'brain failure') affecting higher functions of the brain. There are a number of different recognised causes.

At the time of writing, dementia affects around 850,000 people in the UK, of which Alzheimer's disease (AD) is the commonest cause (62%), followed by vascular dementia (VaD; 17%), dementia with Lewy bodies (DLB; 4%), and frontotemporal dementias, other rarer causes and occasionally reversible conditions (<5%).[1]

These figures include a substantial proportion of cases where there is evidence of mixed pathology – particularly mixtures of Alzheimer's and vascular pathology, which is more common in older people.

The functional domains affected and the evolution of deficits in these domains over time serve as footprints that the clinician can trace back with various levels of certainty to the underlying neuropathology. Definitive classification of dementia is based on the underlying neuropathology, as noted on autopsy or – in rare cases – brain biopsy.

Causes of Alzheimer's disease

Alzheimer's disease is the most common form of dementia. Scientists believe that for most people Alzheimer's disease is caused by a combination of genetic, lifestyle and environmental factors that affect the brain over time.

Early studies using genetic linkage approaches identified familial mutations in proteins related to amyloid-beta production, amyloid precursor protein, presenilin 1 and 2, as well as risk variant apolipoprotein E4. Now, TREM2 variants have been identified as risk factors for Alzheimer's disease and other neurodegenerative diseases.[2]

When neuropathologists examine Alzheimer's disease brain tissue under the microscope, they see two types of abnormalities that are considered hallmarks of the disease: these are amyloid plaques and neurofibrillary tangles. How exactly they contribute to the presentation of disease is an area of long-running discussion.

The amyloid hypothesis

The amyloid hypothesis postulates that the protein amyloid-beta (Aβ) triggers a cascade, harming synapses and ultimately neurons, producing the pathological presentation of Aβ plaques, tau tangles, synapse loss and neurodegeneration, leading to dementia. Aβ accumulation is thought to initiate AD pathology by destroying synapses, causing formation of neurofibrillary tangles, and subsequently resulting in neuron loss.

Secretase enzymes cleave amyloid precursor protein, and problems with this process, specifically mutations in gamma and beta-secretases, can lead to the abnormal production of Aβ. Aβ can then trigger a cascade leading to synaptic damage and neuron loss, and ultimately to the pathological hallmarks of AD: amyloid plaques and neurofibrillary tangles.

But so far, anti-Aβ treatments have broadly failed to meet their primary clinical endpoints when they have been studied and some major phase-three trials of experimental treatments have been halted early. It is also an interesting scientific question why these drugs have failed.

The issues with 'the amyloid hypothesis' are discussed elegantly elsewhere.[3] It is a very major contribution to our understanding of dementia, but it is not without its staunch critics.

Tau hypothesis

Tau is a protein expressed in neurons that normally functions in the stabilisation of microtubules in the cell cytoskeleton. When tau is hyperphosphorylated, this causes it to accumulate into neurofibrillary tangle masses inside nerve cell bodies.

In Alzheimer's disease, threads of hyperphosphorylated tau protein twist into abnormal tangles inside brain cells, leading to failure of the cellular transport system. This failure is also strongly implicated in the decline and death of brain cells.

Causes of vascular dementia

Vascular dementia is caused when the brain's blood supply is interrupted.

Like all organs, the brain needs a constant supply of oxygen and nutrients from the blood to work properly. If the supply of blood is restricted or stopped, then brain cells will begin to die, leading to brain damage and lost function.

If the blood vessels inside the brain narrow and harden, the brain's blood supply can gradually become interrupted. The blood vessels usually narrow and become hard when fatty deposits build up on the blood vessel walls, restricting blood flow. This is called atherosclerosis, and is more common in people who have high blood pressure or type 1 diabetes and those who smoke.

BOX 2.1 CLASSIFICATION AND CAUSES OF SPORADIC VASCULAR COGNITIVE IMPAIRMENT

Post-stroke dementia

Vascular dementia

Multi-infarct dementia (cortical vascular dementia)

Subcortical ischaemic vascular dementia

Strategic-infarct dementia

Hypoperfusion dementia

Haemorrhagic dementia

Dementia caused by specific arteriopathies

Mixed AD and vascular dementia

Vascular mild cognitive impairment

Causes of dementia with Lewy bodies

Lewy bodies are small, circular lumps of protein that develop inside brain cells. It is not known what causes them.

It is currently also unclear how Lewy bodies damage the brain and cause dementia.

It is possible that Lewy bodies interfere with the effects of two of the messenger chemicals in the brain called dopamine and acetylcholine. These messenger chemicals, which send information from one brain cell to another, are called neurotransmitters. Dopamine and acetylcholine are thought to play an important role in regulating brain functions such as memory, learning, mood and attention.

Causes of frontotemporal dementia

In recent years, various genetic factors have been established as important risk factors for frontotemporal dementia (FTD). It is, however, not certain to what extent lifestyle, co-morbidity, environmental factors or cardiovascular risk factors might also have on the overall risk of FTD.

The genetic exploration for understanding common pathological mechanisms involved in neurological diseases is gaining ground. FTD may be associated with motor neuron disease, and the transactive response DNA-binding protein 43 (TDP-43) is a major pathological substrate underlying both diseases.[4] 'Microtubule-associated protein tau' (MAPT), 'granulin' (GRN) and 'chromosome 9 open reading frame72' (C9ORF72) gene mutations are the major known genetic causes of FTD.[5] Recent studies suggest that mutations in these genes may also be associated with other forms of dementia.

In some cases of FTD, the details of genetics, at a molecular level, have allowed some determination of the genotype before the onset of symptoms. In recent years, we have witnessed a new era of molecular genetic understanding of the FTD syndromes.

Different types of dementia and their primary symptoms

Alzheimer's disease

Difficulty learning lists of simple items, or remembering recent conversations, names or events is often an early clinical symptom; apathy and depression are also often early symptoms. Later symptoms include impaired communication, poor judgement, disorientation, confusion, behaviour changes and difficulty speaking, swallowing and walking.

Vascular cognitive impairment

Impaired judgement or ability to make decisions, plan or organise is more likely to be among the initial symptoms, as opposed to the memory loss often associated with the initial symptoms of Alzheimer's. This results from blood vessel blockage or damage leading to infarcts (strokes) or bleeding in the brain. The location, number and size of the brain injury determines how the individual's thinking and physical functioning are affected. Brain imaging can often detect blood vessel problems implicated in vascular dementia.

Dementia with Lewy bodies

Dementia with Lewy bodies (DLB) is a progressive condition which means symptoms get worse over time. The diagnostic criteria for probable DLB currently require at least two of three core features:

- fluctuating attention and concentration

- recurrent well-formed visual hallucinations

- spontaneous Parkinsonian motor signs.

From a cognitive neurology point of view, studies have suggested that memory impairment is less severe in patients with DLB than in those with Alzheimer's disease, while in general there are more severe impairments in visuospatial, attentional and executive abilities. The modest involvement of the temporal lobe fits with the relative preservation of global neuropsychological measures and memory tasks in the early stage of DLB. The selective involvement of parietal, frontal and occipital lobes might explain some of the clinical and neuropsychological features of DLB, providing a possible distinctive marker for this disease.[6]

Lewy bodies are abnormal aggregations (or clumps) of the protein alpha-synuclein. When they develop in a part of the brain called the cortex, dementia can result. Alpha-synuclein also aggregates in the brains of people with Parkinson's disease, but the aggregates may appear in a pattern that is different from DLB.

Mixed dementia

Mixed dementia symptoms may vary, depending on the types of brain changes involved and the brain regions affected. In many cases, symptoms may be similar to or even indistinguishable from those of Alzheimer's or another type of dementia.

Mixed dementia is characterised by the hallmark abnormalities of more than one cause of dementia – most commonly Alzheimer's disease and vascular dementia, but also other types, such as dementia with Lewy bodies.

Parkinson's disease dementia

As Parkinson's disease progresses, it often results in a progressive dementia similar to dementia with Lewy bodies or Alzheimer's disease. Problems with movement are common symptoms of the disease. If dementia develops, symptoms are often similar to dementia with Lewy bodies. Alpha-synuclein clumps are likely to begin in an area deep in the brain called the substantia nigra.

Frontotemporal dementia

Frontotemporal dementia (FTD) is clinically and pathologically heterogeneous.

The recent international consensus papers recognise four main clinical variants – a behavioural variant (bvFTD) characterised by prominent early personality or behavioural changes and three primary progressive aphasia (PPA) syndromes: semantic variant or sv-PPA (previously known as semantic dementia), a non-fluent/agrammatic variant (previously known as progressive non-fluent aphasia) and a logopenic variant.[7] The latter syndrome is distinguished by impairment of lexical retrieval and sentence repetition.

Symptoms tend to reflect where the predominant brain pathology is:

- **Frontal behavioural features**: disinhibition, apathy, loss of empathy, stereotyped or perseverative behaviour, impulsivity, excessive risk taking, alterations in food preferences, executive deficits.

- **Language features**: word-finding difficulties, apraxia of speech, agrammatism, anomia, impaired single-word comprehension, impaired object knowledge, phonologic errors, impaired word/sentence repetition, impaired sentence comprehension, surface dyslexia, dysgraphia.

Posterior cortical atrophy

For some time, there has been a debate whether this is indeed a distinct form of dementia of the Alzheimer type. The term posterior cortical atrophy (PCA) was coined to describe a series of patients with early visual dysfunction in the setting of neurodegeneration of posterior cortical regions. The PCA syndrome aligned with several other reports of patients with similar progressive loss of higher visual function.

People with PCA can often spend a long time before they actually receive their diagnosis. It is not uncommon for people with PCA to first present to opticians with their symptoms.

A classification framework for posterior cortical atrophy has recently been proposed to improve the uniformity of definition of the syndrome in a variety of research settings.[8]

PCA typically presents in the mid-50s or early 60s with a variety of unusual visuoperceptual symptoms, such as diminished ability to interpret, locate or reach for objects under visual guidance; deficits in posterior functions such as maths and writing may also be apparent. Although episodic memory and insight are initially relatively preserved, progression of PCA ultimately leads to a more diffuse pattern of cognitive dysfunction.

The neuroimaging features of PCA are intentionally broad to reflect the loose anatomical description of 'posterior cortical atrophy', with the working group regarding evidence of focal structural (e.g. atrophy on magnetic resonance imaging) or functional (e.g. hypometabolism on ^{18}F-labelled fluorodeoxyglucose positron emission tomography or single-photon emission computed tomography) abnormality in the occipital, parietal and/or occipito-temporo-parietal cortices as supportive of the clinico-radiological syndrome.

Corticobasal degeneration

Corticobasal degeneration (CBD), often also called corticobasal syndrome (CBS), is a rare condition that can cause gradually worsening problems with movement, speech, memory and swallowing. CBD is caused by increasing numbers of brain cells becoming damaged or dying over time.

Most cases of CBD develop in adults aged between 50 and 70. The symptoms of CBD get gradually worse over time. They are very variable and many people only have a few of them.

Symptoms can include:

- a 'clumsy' or 'useless' hand

- 'alien' limb

- rigidity

- complex tremors, limb dystonia, bradykinesia

- problems with balance and coordination

- slow and slurred speech

- symptoms of dementia, such as memory and visual problems

- difficulty swallowing.

One limb is usually affected at first. The rate at which the symptoms progress varies widely from person to person.

CBD occurs when brain cells in certain parts of the brain are damaged as a result of a build-up of a protein called tau.

Creutzfeldt–Jakob disease and variant

CJD is the most common human form of a group of rare, fatal brain disorders affecting people and certain other mammals. Variant CJD ('mad cow disease') occurs in cattle, and has been transmitted to people under certain circumstances.

CJD and its variant can be a rapidly fatal disorder that impairs memory and coordination and causes behaviour changes. Specific CJD symptoms experienced by an individual and the order in which they appear can differ significantly.

Some common features can include:

- depression

- personality changes

- agitation, apathy and mood swings

- rapidly worsening confusion, disorientation and problems with memory, thinking, planning and judgement

- slurred speech

- visual difficulties

- difficulty walking

- muscle stiffness, twitches and involuntary jerky movements.

Prion diseases, such as CJD, occur when abnormal prion protein causes normal prion protein in the brain to fold into the same abnormal shape. How prions 'cascade' in the brain is of enormous research interest.

Electroencephalography (EEG) is an integral part of the diagnostic process in patients with CJD. The EEG has therefore been included in the World Health Organization diagnostic classification criteria of CJD.[9]

This is a very specialist and rare area of dementia. If a person has CJD, the clinical team will pass the information on to the National Congenital Anomaly and Rare Diseases Registration Service.

Normal pressure hydrocephalus

Normal pressure hydrocephalus is a form of communicating hydrocephalus. The term was first coined by Adams and colleagues (1965)[10] to describe hydrocephalus with enlargement of ventricles, normal cerebrospinal fluid (CSF) pressure and a triad of symptoms: gait disturbance, dementia and urinary incontinence.

The syndrome is caused by the build-up of fluid in the brain. Ventriculoperitoneal shunting is the main treatment, with variable success rates.[11]

Huntington's disease

Huntington's disease is a progressive brain disorder caused by a single defective gene on chromosome 4 causing an expanded trinucleotide repeat in the DNA sequence.

Symptoms include abnormal involuntary movements, a severe decline in thinking and reasoning skills, and irritability, depression and other mood changes.

Wernicke–Korsakoff syndrome

Wernicke–Korsakoff syndrome is a chronic memory disorder caused by severe deficiency of thiamine (vitamin B1). Thiamine helps brain cells produce energy from sugar. When thiamine levels fall too low, brain cells cannot generate enough energy to function properly.

Memory problems may be strikingly severe while other thinking and social skills seem relatively unaffected.

The most common cause of this is chronic and heavy alcohol misuse. However, there are many other predisposing factors and causes associated with the condition.[12]

HIV dementia

HIV infection can cause a number of different problems in the functions of the brain. This is known as HIV-associated neurocognitive disorder (HAND). The introduction of combined antiretroviral therapy has dramatically reduced the risk of central nervous system opportunistic infection and severe dementia secondary to HIV infection in the last two decades. However, a milder form of HAND remains prevalent with the introduction of combination antiretroviral therapy having significant impact on quality of life. Cognitive testing remains the 'gold standard' of diagnosis; however, this can be time-consuming. Recently developed screening tools, such as CogState and the revised HIV dementia scale, have very good sensitivity and specificity in the more severe stages of HAND. (Research in this area is relatively young.[13])

Features of dementia that would indicate the need for further assessment

BOX 2.2 NATIONAL OCCUPATIONAL STANDARDS
ON PLANNING ASSESSMENTS

National Occupational Standard SFHCHS38 – 'Plan assessment of an individual's health status' – covers planning and agreeing assessment. The practitioner needs to review referral information, and obtain and review any other relevant information. A decision has to be made, with the individual concerned, on the type of assessment procedure that is to be undertaken, and then steps taken to schedule the procedure.

National Occupational Standard SFHCHS40 – 'Establish a diagnosis of an individual's health condition' – is about determining a diagnosis following initial assessment and investigations of an individual's suspected health condition.

A recommended list of patients who would normally benefit from referral is provided by NHS England in their 2015 document 'Dementia diagnosis and management. A brief pragmatic resource for general practitioners'.[14]

Why early diagnosis of dementia is important and the likely outcomes if assessment and treatment is delayed

'Timely' diagnosis is when the patient wants it *and/or* when care partners need it.

A timely diagnosis of dementia is considered of major importance to ensure adequate access to information, evidence-based treatment, care and support for people with dementia. It opens the door to future care and treatment.

It will help to eliminate the possibility of other, potentially treatable, conditions with dementia-like symptoms being responsible for memory, communication, behaviour and other problems.

It can help people with dementia to make the most of their abilities and potentially benefit from drug and non-drug treatments available. An early diagnosis gives someone the chance to explain to family and friends the changes that are happening, and which can be anticipated to happen, in their life.

Identifying the type of dementia in individuals can help families, care partners and care workers to provide support and to know what to expect.

Subtyping dementia is important to guide treatment and management decisions, particularly dementia with Lewy bodies, Alzheimer's disease and vascular cognitive impairments. Differentiating vascular dementia and Alzheimer's becomes more challenging in older patients and in terms of post-diagnostic support may not significantly influence management.

Making a diagnosis of dementia

A diagnosis of dementia should be made only after a comprehensive assessment that should include history taking, cognitive and mental state examination, physical examination and review of medication, including identification of any drugs that may impair cognitive functioning.

People who are assessed for possible dementia should be asked whether they wish to know the diagnosis if it becomes available and with whom it should be shared. An informant history from somebody close is vital, particularly if the person with probable dementia cannot remember details or has no or little insight into their behavioural or personality changes.

If dementia is mild or questionable, the battery of formal neuropsychological testing is not just focused on memory, but addresses the full range of cognitive functions. At the time of diagnosis, and regularly afterwards, it is necessary to assess medical and psychiatric co-morbidities, including depression and psychosis.

In the clinical cognitive assessment, there is a need to examine attention and concentration orientation, higher-order visual perception, short- and long-term memory, praxis, language and executive function.

Other factors that may affect performance should be taken into account, including educational level, skills, prior level of functioning and attainment, language, sensory impairment, psychiatric illness and physical or neurological problems.

An assessment of dementia with an adult with learning disabilities may be supplemented with an assessment of symptoms. A baseline assessment of adaptive behaviour should be completed with all adults with Down's syndrome.

It is helpful for someone in the practice to be familiar with a couple of cognition tools since it is unrealistic to do anything but a brief 'screen' in a normal primary care consultation. Being able to draw a perfect clock, to all intents and purposes, renders a diagnosis of dementia unlikely.

Brain scans (CT or MRI) are not essential for a clinical diagnosis of dementia. If a scan is justified, detailed clinical information is crucial for the radiologist.

Blood tests rarely contribute to the diagnosis but are needed to rule out underlying pathology and are necessary for Quality and Outcomes Framework (QOF) reporting.[15]

The need for an investigation of signs of dementia with sensitivity and in a way that is appropriate to the person

Proficiency in communication with people living with dementia is recognised to be a key component of person-centred care.

However, communicating with a person living with dementia may be challenging for health and social care professionals, and there is evidence that poor communication contributes to inadequate care of individuals with dementia (IWD) in hospital and community settings.

The diagnosis must be appropriate for the recipient and those closest to him/her at the time of diagnosis, and must be delivered in a way that is appropriate to the individual. In other words, the diagnosis itself should be person-centred too.

The need to appropriately refer patients to access specialist services and support networks

A dementia care plan should be empowering and proactive, written in 'dementia-friendly' language and fully linked in to all aspects of the individual's healthcare record, rather than being a standalone document.

A full person-centred care plan should have core information on demographics, care partner details, information-sharing agreements, admission avoidance, details of other correlated conditions and medication.

A condition-specific care plan – for dementia, for example – would then sit underneath this and include specific goals and actions for how the person with dementia will manage his or her health and wellbeing and the support available to him or her.

Crucial service links/continuity of care: information from other agencies – for example, memory services, dementia advisors, social services and care homes – should be incorporated into the care-planning process through multidisciplinary team working and be reflected in the care plan.

How to differentiate between dementia, delirium, depression and other conditions presenting with similar symptoms

Delirium

Delirium is an acute, severe neuropsychiatric syndrome seen mainly in older people in hospital and associated with increased morbidity and mortality. It is common, serious and represents a medical emergency. There have been successful recent initiatives to make all clinicians aware of the existence of delirium in their patients.[16]

The condition causes significant distress and is associated with poor outcomes including increased risk of dementia, death, long-term care admission and length of hospital stay.

People admitted to hospital or a care home who are at risk of delirium should be assessed and given support and treatment to reduce their risk. The care and treatment of patients with delirium needs a multidisciplinary and person-centred approach.

Needs such as pain, hunger, thirst and sensory aids should be identified and addressed, while staff should adopt a reassuring approach, incorporating effective communication and reorientation.

Features that help differentiate delirium and dementia include rapid onset, short duration and disturbance of the level of conscious awareness that often waxes and wanes between agitation and lethargy. People with dementia are at increased risk of developing delirium, and therefore any sudden change in their abilities or behaviour should be investigated so that delirium can be excluded.

Delirium may conceivably be distinguished from dementia by virtue of the disproportionate impairment of vigilance and attention.

Dementia is the strongest risk factor for developing delirium, with delirium superimposed on dementia accounting for many delirium cases in hospital. Differentiating delirium superimposed on dementia from diffuse Lewy body disease (DLB) or delirium alone is vital to guide initial management and safe prescribing.

Delirium is associated with worsening of dementia and is a risk factor for subsequent dementia, with only 19 per cent of people with delirium free from cognitive deficits three months later.[17]

Incorrectly diagnosing an acute change as a deterioration in patients with existing DLB rather than delirium can result in the under-investigation of common causes of delirium, such as infections, medications and pain, and inadequate management of this potentially life-threatening medical emergency.

Conversely, the lack of recognition of undiagnosed DLB in someone with delirium may result in patients being treated with antipsychotic medications and the risk of harmful side effects.

Key is identifying *those most at risk*. Risk factors are: age over 65 years, cognitive impairment or dementia, hip fracture and severe illness.

Measures to prevent delirium include:

- providing frequent orientation (e.g. using clocks and calendars)

- ensuring adequate hydration and nutrition

- detecting and treating pain, constipation and infection

- reviewing medication and avoiding delirogenic drugs

- reducing noise and avoiding interventions during sleep periods

- cognitive stimulation (e.g. playing cards and doing puzzles).

Delirium has a number of possible causes and, in many cases, two or more factors contribute to it. Identifying the cause is important, as treating it may reverse the delirium. Causes include infection, constipation, dehydration, change of environment, acute metabolic disturbance, trauma, hypoxia and alcohol or drug withdrawal.

Delirium can sometimes be the only symptom of a serious underlying disease. Its serious nature means it is vital that professionals working with older people or those with long-term conditions know the main features of delirium to ensure that further assessment and treatment can be organised promptly. This is particularly the case for people with dementia, who are at increased risk of delirium.

Signs and symptoms of delirium include impaired attention, memory disturbance, disorientation and disorganised thinking, altered perceptions (visual hallucinations, illusions, delusions) and emotional disturbance.

One of the key features of delirium is the onset of symptoms being associated with the presence of a physical illness. The main focus of the management of delirium is to find, and treat, the underlying cause. If delirium is suspected, it is important for the patient to have a full physical examination, blood tests and other investigations.

Depression

Depression is common in older people and is generally under-detected and under-diagnosed. In older people its symptoms can be slightly different from those typical for younger adults. For example, older people may experience more physical symptoms and increased anxiety or agitation.

Sleep disturbance is also common, and is a risk factor for depression in this group.

There is a higher risk of suicide among older people with depression.

Depression is a broad diagnosis in which low mood and/or loss of interest or pleasure in most activities are key features.

Various assessment tools are available, and staff should select one that is appropriate and validated. Assessment should be person-centred, seeking symptoms of depression, and a useful mnemonic is 'SIGECAMPS'.[18]

BOX 2.3 'SIGECAMPS'

S – **S**leep disturbance

I – Loss of **I**nterest or pleasure in usual activities

G – Excessive feelings of **G**uilt or worthlessness

E – Decreased **E**nergy and increased fatigue

C – Diminished ability to think or **C**oncentrate

A – **A**ppetite change with weight loss/gain

M – **M**ood is low most days

P – **P**sychomotor agitation or retardation

S – **S**uicidal ideation

It is also important to review briefly suicide risk factors (e.g. older, male sex, widowed, losses, loneliness, medical illness, previous self-harm). It is therefore also important to enquire about past psychiatric history, past medical history, medications and substances, family history and personal history, and not focus solely on symptoms but also on the degree of difficulty with daily living the person is experiencing, and the impact of the suspected depression.

A comprehensive assessment for dementia utilising appropriate investigations and tools

It can be difficult for health professionals to assess accurately cognitive function in older people. Yet this is one of the most important assessments clinicians make, particularly those working in old-age psychiatry and geriatric medicine. It is essential to detecting and diagnosing dementia.

There are a number of assessment scales available but none of them cover this broad range of use. In addition, some scales have a cost attached to them which hinders their use in clinical practice. This includes the widely used Mini Mental State Examination (MMSE).

Cognitive assessments cover a very broad range of activities. They can take place:

- **in a number of settings** – primary care, specialist memory clinics, acute care and care homes

- **for a variety of purposes** – screening, diagnosing, staging and measuring change

- **over a number of domains** – memory, language, visuospatial ability and executive function.[19]

Possible recommended cognitive assessment tools are shown below.

BOX 2.4 SOME ASSESSMENT TOOLS[20]

Primary care

Abbreviated mental test score (AMTS)

General practitioner assessment of cognition (GPCOG)

Mini-cog

Memory clinics

Addenbrookes cognitive examination-III (ACE-III)

Montreal cognitive assessment (MoCA)

Mini mental state examination (MMSE) (Copyright restrictions apply)

Acute care settings

Abbreviated mental test score (AMTS)

6-item cognitive impairment test (6CIT)

General practitioner assessment of cognition (GPCOG)

Care homes

Abbreviated mental test score (AMTS)

6-item cognitive impairment test (6CIT)

General practitioner assessment of cognition (GPCOG)

Montreal cognitive assessment (MoCA)

A differential diagnosis of dementia and the underlying disease processes, where appropriate to clinical role

Diagnosing dementia is a two-stage process.

The first stage is to establish a diagnosis of dementia and the second is to elucidate the cause of the dementia.

When assessing someone who has memory problems, it is important for the clinician to remember that not all people with memory problems have dementia. There are several conditions which mimic dementia and can be easily missed if the clinician is not actively looking for them.

The main 'three Ds' of differential diagnoses/potential contributing factors are summarised thus:[21]

- **Depression**: this may be contributing to the presentation in a patient with dementia.

- **Drugs**: for example, those with strong anticholinergic activity, such as tricyclic antidepressants, older drugs for bladder problems and first-generation antihistamines, should be stopped if possible or substituted for a drug with less anticholinergic activity.

- **Delirium**: the diagnosis should be clear from the timescale and the general condition of the patient.

The potential impact of diagnostic errors

Diagnosis is one of the most important tasks performed by primary care physicians. The World Health Organization has prioritised patient safety areas in primary care and included diagnostic errors as a high-priority problem.

In addition, a report from the Institute of Medicine in the USA, *Improving Diagnosis in Health Care*, published in 2015, concluded that most people will likely experience a diagnostic error in their lifetime.

Several studies have suggested that symptom severity and degree of impairment are important predictors of diagnostic sensitivity. Since patients with early dementia are most likely to benefit from intervention, future efforts to improve the timeliness of dementia diagnosis should especially focus on detection of more subtle and early manifestations of the disease.

The experience of a person with dementia and their family and care partners must involve sensitive communication about the diagnosis of dementia and related implications

A diagnosis is often regarded by those with dementia and family members as a positive and constructive event, particularly when any initial shock has worn off.

Critically, the response to a diagnosis depends on how a person with dementia is told about it – and the level of support that is available to them and their families after diagnosis. It is therefore important for the person with dementia and their family to receive the dementia diagnosis in a positive way, with time made available to answer any questions and for support and reassurance to be provided.

This is more likely to lead to the individual feeling more in control and empowered to make decisions.

The particular impact of a diagnosis for younger people with dementia and their families

In terms of young-onset dementia (people under 65), the Alzheimer's Society estimates that there are over 40,000 younger people with dementia in the UK.[22] This equates to 5 per cent of all people with dementia. This is an important consideration for organisations providing care and support services.

Research suggests that young people caring for a loved one with dementia provide a range of practical, emotional and social support. However, in common with many children and young people supporting individuals with other conditions, some do not identify themselves as 'young care partners' or feel comfortable with the label.

The available literature describes a range of challenges and issues for young people living with a person with dementia:

- strain on relationships with the person with dementia and other family members (and related themes of problems in adaptation and coping)

- impact on education, employment and other future plans

- a lack of professional and public awareness of young people's needs and experiences, and therefore of age-appropriate and relevant support.

The needs of people with learning disabilities and dementia

A person with a learning disability may have already behaved in ways that are considered to reflect distress and this can worsen if they develop dementia. The person may have a different sense of reality because of the dementia. By understanding this, care partners can begin to be aware of what they might be feeling, and be able to interpret their behaviour.

Care partners and professionals should work together to understand the reasons or triggers for the person's behaviour and ways of preventing it.

A person with a learning disability and dementia may be able to continue with many activities for some time if they are given the right support. He/she should be encouraged to maintain his/her independence for as long as possible, if he/she desires it.

All interventions and management plans need to have the person as the centre of focus and this will therefore require a holistic approach that takes into account the person's expressed views.

Treatment and support for other conditions more common in people with Down's syndrome (e.g. hearing loss, depression, seizures, underactive thyroid) may be made more complicated by the person's dementia.

The importance of equal access to dementia assessment and diagnosis for people from diverse communities

People with dementia and their care partners should always be treated with the utmost respect. People with dementia should not be excluded from services because of their diagnosis, age (whether regarded as too old or too young) or any learning disability.

If there is a language barrier, they should be offered:

- written information in the preferred language and/or an accessible format

- interpreters

- psychological interventions in the preferred language.

People suspected of having dementia because of cognitive and functional deterioration, but who do not have sufficient overall functional impairment for diagnosis, should not be denied access to support services.

The delivery of care and support that is in line with the needs and wants of the individual is critical to ensure that the person receives personalised care and support. A person's culture and background are clearly significant components of their identity.

Black and minority ethnic (BAME) people are generally under-represented in dementia services, and the development of appropriate health and social care services to meet their needs has been a long-standing policy priority.

Lower levels of awareness about dementia and the existence of stigma within BAME communities help to explain some of the reasons why BAME people are currently under-represented in dementia services. However, staff can adopt several approaches to improving the uptake of services, such as developing different information resources and appointing workers with responsibility for outreach.

Care partners of BAME people with dementia may feel reluctant to ask for help, although support in the form of care partners' groups and respite services may be appreciated.

The need to document assessment and diagnosis decisions

When a physician makes the diagnosis of dementia, it is very important that they discuss the diagnosis with the patient (where appropriate) and with their care partners, and document that this discussion has taken place.

A new diagnosis of dementia must always be communicated to the patient's GP.

Notes

1. Alzheimer's Society, 'Demography.' Accessed on 2 October 2017 at www.alzheimers.org.uk/info/20091/what_we_think/93/demography

2. Jay, T.R., von Saucken, V. and Landreth, G.E. (2017) 'TREM2 in Neurodegenerative Diseases.' *Molecular Neurodegeneration 12*, 1, 56.

3. Morris, G.P., Clark, I.A. and Vissel, B. (2014) 'Inconsistencies and controversies surrounding the amyloid hypothesis of Alzheimer's disease.' *Acta Neuropathologica Communications 18*, 2, 135.

4. Couratier, P., Corcia, P., Lautrette, G., Nicol, M. and Marin, B. (2017) 'ALS and frontotemporal dementia belong to a common disease spectrum.' *Revue Neurologique (Paris) 173*, 5, 273–279.

5. Guven, G., Lohmann, E., Bras, J., Gibbs, J.R. *et al.* (2016) 'Mutation frequency of the major frontotemporal dementia genes, MAPT, GRN and C9ORF72 in a Turkish cohort of dementia patients.' *PLoS One 11*, 9, e0162592. Accessed on 2 October 2017 at http://journals.plos.org/plosone/article?id=10.1371/journal.pone.0162592

6. Bozzali, M., Falini, A., Cercignani, M., Baglio, F. *et al.* (2005) 'Brain tissue damage in dementia with Lewy bodies: An in vivo diffusion tensor MRI study.' *Brain 128*, Pt 7, 1595–1604.

7. Bott, N.T., Radke, A., Stephens, M.L. and Kramer, J.H. (2014) 'Frontotemporal dementia: diagnosis, deficits and management.' *Neurodegener Dis Manag 4*, 6, 439–454. Accessed on 6 November 2017 at www.ncbi.nlm.nih.gov/pmc/articles/PMC4824317

8. Crutch, S.J., Schott, J.M., Rabinovici, G.D., Murray, M. *et al.* (2017) 'Consensus classification of posterior cortical atrophy.' *Alzheimers and Dementia: The Journal of the Alzheimer's Association 13*, 8, 870–884.

9. Wieser, H.G., Schindler, K. and Zumsteg, D. (2006) *Clinical Neurophysiology 117*, 5, 935–951. Accessed on 2 October 2017 at www.clinph-journal.com/article/S1388-2457(05)00511-0/abstract

10. Adams R.D., Fisher C.M., Hakim S., Ojemann R.G. and Sweet W.H. (1965) 'Symptomatic occult hydrocephalus with "normal" cerebrospinal fluid pressure: A treatable syndrome.' *New England Journal of Medicine 27*, 117–126.

11. Nassar, B.R. and Lippa, C.F. (2016) 'Idiopathic normal pressure hydrocephalus.' *Gerontology and Geriatric Medicine 2*. Accessed on 2 October 2017 at www.ncbi.nlm.nih.gov/pmc/articles/PMC5119812/#bibr1-2333721416643702

12. Donnelly, A. (2017) 'Wernicke-Korsakoff syndrome: Recognition and treatment.' *Nursing Standard 31*, 31, 46–53.

13. Carroll, A. and Brew, B. (2017) 'HIV-associated neurocognitive disorders: Recent advances in pathogenesis, biomarkers, and treatment.' *F1000Research*. Accessed on 2 October 2017 at https://f1000research.com/articles/6-312/v1; Brew, B.J. and Chan, P. (2014) 'Update on HIV dementia and HIV-associated neurocognitive disorders.' *Current Neurology and Neuroscience Reports* https://www.england.nhs.uk/wp-content/uploads/2015/01/dementia-diag-mng-ab-pt.pdf *14*, 8, 468.

14. Accessed on 2 October 2017 at www.england.nhs.uk/wp-content/uploads/2015/01/dementia-diag-mng-ab-pt.pdf

15. NHS England (2015) 'Dementia diagnosis and management: A brief pragmatic resource for general practitioners', p.6. Accessed on 2 October 2017 at www.england.nhs.uk/wp-content/uploads/2015/01/dementia-diag-mng-ab-pt.pdf

16. For example, Commissioning for Quality and Innovation (CQUIN): https://www.england.nhs.uk/wp-content/uploads/2015/03/9-cquin-guid-2015-16.pdf

17. Jackson, T.A., Gladman, J.R., Harwood, R.H., MacLullich, A.M. *et al.* (2017) 'Challenges and opportunities in understanding dementia and delirium in the acute hospital.' *PLoS Medicine 14*, 3, e1002247.

18. BMJ (2006) 'A mnemonic for depression.' Accessed on 1 September 2017 at www.bmj.com/rapid-response/2011/10/31/mnemonic-depression

19. Alzheimer's Society (2013) 'Helping you to assess cognition. A practical toolkit for clinicians.' Accessed on 1 September 2017 at http://oxleas.nhs.uk/site-media/cms-downloads/AS_Cognitive_Assessment_Toolkit.pdf

20. Derived from Alzheimer's Society (2013) 'Helping you to assess cognition. A practical toolkit for clinicians.'

21. NHS England (2015) 'Dementia diagnosis and management: A brief pragmatic resource for general practitioners', pp.10–11. Accessed on 2 October 2017 at www.england.nhs.uk/wp-content/uploads/2015/01/dementia-diag-mng-ab-pt.pdf.

22. Alzheimer's Society (2017) 'Facts for the media.' Accessed on 1 September 2017 at www.alzheimers.org.uk/info/20027/news_and_media/541/facts_for_the_media

3

Dementia risk reduction and prevention

Dementia imposes a huge emotional and financial cost, but people living with dementia and their care partners have capacity to bring enormous value to society.

As yet there are no therapies that delay or slow the progression of the condition. There is, however, a general consensus that public health and dementia prevention need to form part of the agenda.

It is agreed that dementia risk reduction and prediction are a critical part of 'dementia awareness'. There needs to be greater awareness of the lifestyle issues that may increase the risk of dementia and an emphasis given to the fact that people need to pay greater attention to their own health and how they can help prevent or reduce the risk of the onset of dementia.

It has been suggested that up to 30 per cent of Alzheimer's disease and dementia cases more broadly may be preventable through modifiable health and lifestyle factors.[1]

Directly or indirectly, dementia will soon affect every one of us. Dementia is the most feared health condition for people over the age of 55 according to a survey by Alzheimer's Research UK. Dementia is more feared than any other major disease, including cancer and diabetes.[2]

As the number of people with dementia rises, so too do the associated healthcare costs. It is hoped that dementia risk reduction will save the health and social care system money by reducing the prevalence and impact of dementia across the population and support people to live longer, healthier lives.

The benefits of dementia prevention reach far beyond the health and social care system. It is, however, well recognised that dementia is a complex, multifactorial condition, with risk factors asserting varying influences throughout the life course.

Lifestyle factors that may increase the risk of developing certain types of dementia

The scientific evidence is evolving rapidly and is already sufficient to justify considered action and further research on dementia risk reduction, both by reducing the modifiable risk factors and improving the recognised protective factors.

Given the evidence that there may be a vascular component to many dementias, interventions to address vascular risk factors could also help reduce the risk, progression and severity of dementia.

These include tobacco smoking, eating a poor diet high in saturated fat, sugar and salt, obesity in midlife, a lack of regular physical activity along with a sedentary lifestyle and excessive alcohol consumption, and intermediate disease precursors such as raised blood pressure, raised blood cholesterol and diabetes which arise from behavioural and other factors.

Protective factors also play a part and these include education and intellectual and social engagement.

Lifestyle changes may delay the onset and severity of certain types of dementia

At this time, it is not possible to either prevent or cure dementia, although there is extensive research in both areas.

It is appropriate, however, to consider ways of reducing the risk of developing dementia with the hope that such approaches may either delay or prevent onset or severity. Indeed, a few studies have suggested that the age-specific incidence of dementia (i.e. the risk of dementia at any specific age) might be decreasing.[3]

A substantial proportion of dementia might be delayed or averted if modifiable risk factors are effectively addressed.

A life-course approach to the study of dementia supports the notion that certain risk factors may operate at critical periods with varying strength of association observed at different time periods.

Brain and cognitive reserve, developed early in life and consolidated in midlife, may buffer the expression of symptoms of dementia in the presence of neurodegenerative disease. This leads to the mantra 'use it or lose it'.

Early-life growth and development, higher educational achievement, mentally stimulating activity, social engagement and physical exercise may all contribute to this process, and help to ward off the development and clinical manifestations of dementia in later life.

Vascular risk factors (i.e. high blood pressure, cholesterol, diabetes and obesity) become more prevalent in midlife, and are plausibly linked to risk for dementia through a variety of cerebrovascular disease, inflammatory and neurodegenerative pathways.

Cognitive decline and dementia are multicausal

The most common cause of dementia is Alzheimer's disease. Vascular dementia is the second most common type of dementia, affecting around 150,000 people in the UK.[4]

However, there is increasing evidence that individual cases of dementia are often a mixture of Alzheimer's disease and vascular dementia. Vascular dementia has the same risk factors as cardiovascular disease and stroke, and so the same preventive measures are likely to reduce risk.

Age is the biggest risk factor for dementia. This increased risk may be due to factors associated with ageing, such as:

- higher blood pressure in midlife

- an increased incidence of some diseases

- cellular mechanisms of 'senescence'

- changes in the immune system.

It has been argued that many of the published trials in dementia have considered the impact of a single intervention on a single risk factor, which is overly simplistic.

The recent interim results from the FINGER study demonstrate that it is possible to have, albeit very modest, impact on cognitive decline through reductions in multiple risk factors.[5]

Without controlled, interventional studies, it is not possible to infer causality from risk factor associations and to know therefore whether lifestyle and behavioural modification can reduce the incidence or delay the onset of dementia.

Other actions which may reduce risks for dementia more directly could include known factors such as reducing alcohol and substance abuse and preventing head injuries, particularly in young people.

The impact in early life of these and other risk factors (including maternal health and behaviours and parental skills, physical activity levels, etc.) and protective factors (including educational attainment) should be urgently examined from a policy and research perspective.

Dementia risk reduction evidence-based research

Determining the relative contributions of the risk factors to different forms of dementia is a research priority, and the role of some factors (e.g. alcohol intake), and their interaction with genetic characteristics, is still being explored.

Notwithstanding this, the global increases in Alzheimer's disease and other dementias, and the observed associations with modifiable factors, have prompted researchers and advocates to recommend that population-level risk-reduction strategies be instigated by government and non-government agencies.

A growing number of organisations are heeding this call, demonstrated by initiatives such as the Healthy Brain Initiative in the US, the Your Brain Matters campaign in Australia, the National Memory Programme in Finland and the Forget Me Not education programme in Ireland.[6]

This new arena of evidence-based research has brought with it a need for new evidence about the prevailing knowledge, beliefs and behaviours concerning dementia and the potential to maintain cognitive health among different population segments.

Approaches to 'evidence'

The *Oxford English Dictionary* states that evidence comprises 'information or signs indicating whether a belief or proposition is true or valid', from the Old French/Latin *evidentia*, 'obvious to the mind or eye'.[7]

- **Evidence-based healthcare** is the conscientious use of current best evidence in making decisions about the care of individual patients or the delivery of health services.

- **Evidence-based clinical practice** is an approach to decision-making in which the clinician uses the best evidence available, in consultation with the patient, to decide upon the option which suits that patient best.

- **Evidence-based medicine** is the conscientious, explicit and judicious use of current best evidence in making decisions about the care of individual patients.

Future prevalence estimates highlight the need for urgent intervention focused on risk reduction because even a modest delay in onset can result in significant public health gains.

Dementia research is largely focused on areas in which those investing have judged that there will be greatest return on that investment and highest impact. However, a parallel strategy is needed to address this societal problem.

A new approach tackling other dimensions is required including:

- identifying new risk factors for dementia through research into the mechanisms for the development and progression of dementia

- epidemiological studies to understand the importance of risk factors in the development of dementia, particularly in early and midlife

- epidemiological and modelling studies to help describe and predict the burdens of dementia in the UK population and the potential returns on investment that will accrue from prevention policies

- follow-up of existing trials and cohort studies – such as those for diabetes and cardiovascular disease – to examine long-term implications on dementia outcomes.

Health promotion

Health promotion has been considered relevant by policy makers to cope successfully with ageing populations and respective health problems, and thus has become an integral part of the healthy and active ageing policy.

There is positive movement towards these ends in initiatives such as the UK Dementia Platform[8] and the EU Joint Programme on Neurodegenerative Disorders.[9]

There is persuasive evidence that the dementia risk for populations can be modified through reduction in tobacco use and better control and detection for hypertension and diabetes, as well as cardiovascular risk factors.

A good (and accurate) mantra is 'What is good for your heart is good for your brain.'

This is supported by current national guidance on midlife approaches to delay or prevent the onset of dementia, disability and frailty in later life from the National Institute for Health and Care Excellence (NICE).[10]

A major study published in *The Lancet Neurology*[11] found that around a third of Alzheimer's disease cases worldwide might be attributable to potentially modifiable risk factors. The study found that, in the UK, physical activity was estimated to have the greatest influence of the risk factors studied. The study found also that Alzheimer's disease in 21.8 per cent of people was estimated to be attributable to physical inactivity. This proportion arguably could potentially be prevented if people were more active in older age.[12]

Keeping one's brain active and challenged throughout life may help reduce the risk of dementia. Research shows that a lower risk of developing dementia is associated with:

- higher levels of education

- more mentally demanding occupations

- cognitive stimulation, such as doing puzzles or learning a second language.

A further review[13] of brain reserve and cognitive decline, combining the data from 22 studies and more than 29,000 participants, found a 46 per cent lower risk of dementia in those with high levels of mental activity than those with low mental activity. Being socially active might help to reduce dementia risk by:

- improving your mood

- relieving stress

- reducing the risk of depression

- reducing loneliness.

Introduction to national health promotion strategies

Previous work suggests that there are three models of health education – preventive, radical-political and self-empowerment – each of which describes a different role for information campaigns in the process of behaviour change.

The preventive model focuses on individuals and the use of education to motivate healthy decisions and encourage people to behave in a healthy way.

According to the Ottawa Charter for Health Promotion,[14] health promotion can be described as follows:

> Health promotion is the process of enabling people to increase control over, and to improve, their health. To reach a state of complete physical, mental and social well-being, an individual or group must be able to identify and to realize aspirations, to satisfy needs, and to change or cope with the environment. Health is, therefore, seen as a resource for everyday life, not the objective of living. Health is a positive concept emphasizing social and personal resources, as well as physical capacities. Therefore, health promotion is not just the responsibility of the health sector, but goes beyond healthy life-styles to well-being.

Smoking cessation and improved detection and treatment of diabetes and hypertension should be prioritised, including for older adults who are rarely specifically targeted in prevention programmes. Increased physical activity and reduction in levels of obesity are also important.

The Blackfriars Consensus on promoting brain health was developed after a meeting in London in January 2014, hosted by the UK Health Forum and Public Health England (PHE), and is supported by 60 experts and organisations in dementia and non-communicable diseases (NCD) prevention.[15] It was a powerful and significant contribution.

Dementia risk reduction should begin to be incorporated into both national and global policies to tackle NCDs, beginning with the interventions where the evidence is most robust, but recognising that this will be likely to evolve rapidly.

Evidence-based health promotion involves the systematic integration of research evidence into the planning and implementation of health promotion activities.

The NHS Health Check,[16] for adults in England aged 40 to 74, is an ideal opportunity for GPs and other healthcare professionals to offer advice to promote a healthier lifestyle. It also offers an opportunity to take regular measurements of cholesterol levels, blood glucose and blood pressure.

It is common in midlife to have one or more of the seven health risk factors identified by the Chief Medical Officer:[17]

1. smoking

2. binge drinking

3. low fruit and vegetable consumption

4. obesity

5. diabetes

6. high blood pressure

7. raised cholesterol.

The NHS Health Check includes a dementia component which aims to increase awareness of dementia among people aged 65 to 74.

Clinical commissioning groups (CCGs) can play a key role in promoting dementia risk reduction. To do this they need access to high-quality and relevant dementia data. PHE's Dementia Intelligence Network has launched the first dementia profile.[18] This is a tool that enables bespoke comparison and benchmarking for local authorities and CCGs against other areas in England using one, easily accessible online platform.

CCGs could use the data to look at local risk factors for dementia such as smoking prevalence, physical inactivity, excess weight and alcohol-related hospital admissions.

The NICE guideline on midlife approaches to delay or prevent the onset of dementia, disability and frailty in later life[19] recommends a major role for local government and Health and Wellbeing Boards.

Stronger collaboration between clinical practitioners, public health and prevention experts, researchers and policy makers concerned with dementia or with other NCDs is needed to support better integration of policy development and more effective programme implementation and evaluation. There is also an urgent need for research in implementation science to inform such approaches.

Motivational factors that may have an impact on the ability to make changes

---

BOX 3.1 NATIONAL OCCUPATIONAL STANDARDS ON ENCOURAGING BEHAVIOURAL CHANGE

National Occupational Standard SFHPHP15 – 'Encourage behavioural change in people and agencies to promote health and wellbeing' – covers encouraging behaviour change in people and agencies in order to promote health and wellbeing. This includes the three stages of: enabling people and agencies to see the need for and to change their behaviour; enabling people to sustain their behaviour change; and evaluating the effectiveness of behaviour change.

There is a large body of theoretical work that has sought to explain the determinants of human behaviour.

Health behaviour theory

Health behaviour theory has a plethora of theoretical constructs, which are often very similar or indeed identical to each other but use different terminology. Attempts have been made to develop an integrated theory and to distil similar concepts from these different theories.

There are many different ideas about what factors affect whether someone will change (and maintain) lifestyle behaviours.

Most of the main theories include a concept relating to confidence (i.e. belief in one's ability to perform the behaviour) and to motivation (i.e. one's desire or will to engage in the behaviour).

People need enough knowledge of potential dangers to warrant action, but they do not have to be scared out of their wits to act.

The term 'motivation' is used to refer both to our reasons for action (*What is your motive?*) and to our enthusiasm for doing it (*How motivated are you?*).

Under the 'health belief model', behaviour change requires a state of readiness to act. This state is affected by an individual's perceptions about their personal susceptibility to a particular health condition and whether the consequences are perceived to be serious.

Information campaigns can play a major role in behaviour change. It is suggested that they should emphasise personal susceptibility and the seriousness of not making a change, and should outline the costs of unhealthy behaviours and the benefits of change.

Social cognitive theory

Social cognitive theory incorporates the basic components of social learning theory but adds the principles of observational learning and vicarious reinforcement (watching and learning from the actions of others).

As an individual adopts new behaviour, this causes changes in both the environment and the individual. According to this theory, self-efficacy is considered the most important personal factor in behaviour change.

The main features are depicted in Figure 3.1.

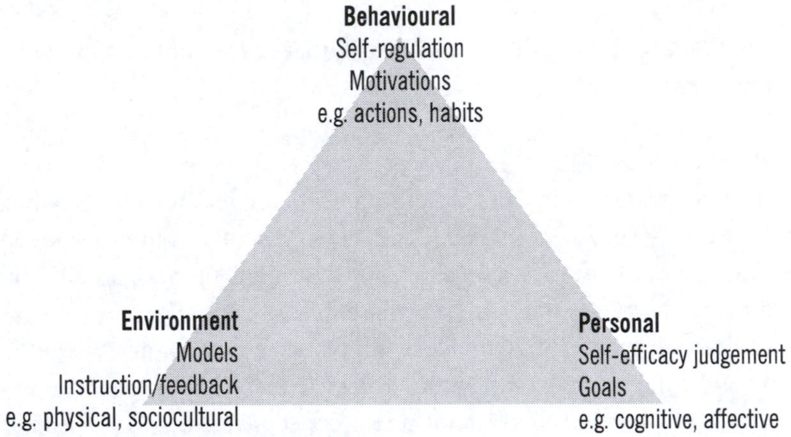

Behavioural
Self-regulation
Motivations
e.g. actions, habits

Environment
Models
Instruction/feedback
e.g. physical, sociocultural

Personal
Self-efficacy judgement
Goals
e.g. cognitive, affective

Figure 3.1 Social cognitive theory

Signposting to sources of health promotion information and support

Under the theory of planned behaviour, a successful behaviour-change intervention must do more than pass on information about the costs and benefits of a behaviour and should inspire a feeling of personal susceptibility. In order for information to influence behaviour, it would also have to tackle perceived normative beliefs. It should make someone believe the healthy behaviour is 'normal'.

This might involve, for example, using mass media channels to plant storylines in soap operas such as *Emmerdale*, or getting celebrities or likable characters to convey a message, making it appear the 'cool' thing to be interested in (e.g. famous actors or comedians with their own life experience of dementia).

Following a diagnosis of dementia, it is worth making time available to discuss the diagnosis with the person with dementia and, if the person consents, with their family. Both may need ongoing support.

Any advice and information given should be documented in the notes.

Communicating effectively messages about healthy living according to the abilities and needs of individuals

---

BOX 3.2 NATIONAL OCCUPATIONAL STANDARDS ON COMMUNICATION

National Occupations Standard SFHHT2 – 'Communicate with individuals about promoting their health and wellbeing' – is about communicating to promote the development of healthy behaviours and lifestyles to improve health and wellbeing.

Communication theory holds that multi-level strategies are necessary depending on who is being targeted, such as tailored messages at the individual level, targeted messages at the group level, social marketing at the community level, media advocacy at the policy level and mass media campaigns at the population level.

The general public, health professionals and policy makers are increasingly aware of the links between behavioural risk factors and non-communicable diseases (such as tobacco and lung cancer or diet and cardiovascular disease). But few people are aware that many of the same risk factors could impact on the risk of dementia.

Efforts to encourage people to adopt health practices rely heavily on persuasive communications in health education campaigns.

In such health messages, appeals to fear by depicting the ravages of disease like a 'shrinking orange' are often used as motivators, and the level of fear elicited in such a message should only be such to elicit a desired behaviour (such as avoiding risk factors for dementia, or donating money to a dementia charity).[20]

It is therefore important to communicate more clearly the emerging evidence about dementia risks, protective factors and preventive actions to the public and relevant health and care professionals and policy makers.

Further population-based work on the impact of dementia awareness and risk messaging is important in order to assess its contribution to perceptions of stigma and fear, as well as potential to change behaviour at the individual level. This will influence the balance of preventive strategies.

Communications should continue to tackle the myths and misinformation about dementia and to reduce stigma, and should be carefully framed to avoid the impression that individuals who develop dementia are to blame through insufficient adherence to perceived preventive behaviours.

Lessons learned from the experience of communicating the risks of other non-communicable diseases such as cancer may be valuable.

Developing and disseminating health promotion information and advice

---

BOX 3.3 NATIONAL OCCUPATIONAL STANDARDS ON DISSEMINATING INFORMATION

National Occupational Standard SCDHSC0438 – 'Develop and disseminate information and advice about health and social well-being' – identifies the requirements when developing a range of information and advice materials to promote services and raise awareness of health and social wellbeing. The requirements include planning, design, production and dissemination of information and advice materials.

National Occupational Standard SCDHSC0438 – 'Develop and disseminate information and advice about health and social well-being' – evaluates the production and dissemination of information and advice materials. It suggests important quality markers, such as needs to (1) identify the overall purpose of the information and advice materials and specific objectives to be achieved through their dissemination, (2) monitor the process of design, production and dissemination, (3) establish criteria for evaluating the effectiveness of information and advice materials in achieving the original objective, and (4) collect and review information on the effectiveness of information and advice materials in achieving the original objectives.

Accuracy is a cornerstone of good-quality health information, so it is essential that information is based on thorough research and sound evidence. Signposting to further information and support will help to give a balanced picture, without overloading the reader with too much information. Clear and simple language suited to the target group is fundamental to effective communication.

In providing health information, consideration must be given to all potential users in the target audience, including ethnic minority groups, people with disabilities and those whose first language is not English.

This is not simply a language issue – it has implications for the presentation of information, its format and the channels of distribution.

It is worth identifying when it is appropriate for design and production to be contracted to media professionals, and when it might be necessary to provide any media professionals involved in design or production with a detailed briefing.

Dissemination of information and advice materials

Dissemination means more than compiling a mailing list. In order to ensure effective use of information, careful planning must take place regarding the way it is used, by whom and for what purpose. These elements will have significant implications for the training and professional development of intermediary users.

Targeted dissemination systems must be in place across organisations to check that the process for reaching the target groups is effective. The process must be reviewed regularly to ensure that systems are updated.

Encouraging behavioural change in individuals and organisations

There are various models of behavioural change in health promotion. The acceptance of one's susceptibility to a disease that is also believed to be serious provides a force leading to action, but it does not define the particular course of action that is likely to be taken.

The direction that the action will take is influenced by beliefs regarding the relative effectiveness of known available alternatives in reducing the disease threat to which the individual feels subjected.

Box 3.4 shows some examples of behavioural change models.

BOX 3.4 DIFFERENT MODELS FOR BEHAVIOURAL CHANGE
Health belief model

This model proposes that people, when presented with a risk message, engage in two appraisal processes: a determination of whether they are susceptible to an identified threat and whether the threat is severe; and whether the recommended action can reduce that threat (i.e. response efficacy) and whether they can successfully perform the recommended action.

The trans-theoretical model of change

Behaviour change is viewed as a progression through a series of five stages: pre-contemplation, contemplation, preparation, action and maintenance.

Theory of planned behaviour

This theory holds that intent is influenced not only by the attitude towards behaviour but also the perception of social norms (the strength of others' opinions on the behaviour and a person's own motivation to comply with those of significant others) and the degree of perceived behavioural control.

Activated health model

This is a three-phase model that actively engages individuals in the assessment of their health (experiential phase); presents information and creates awareness of the target behaviour (awareness phase); and facilitates its identification and clarification of personal health values, and develops a customised plan for behaviour change (responsibility phase).

Policies for dementia prevention should include upstream population-level actions as well as community- and individual-level interventions. Personalised interventions to encourage behaviour change, such as education and awareness campaigns, could need to be supported by upstream policies such as regulating and taxing health-damaging products.

The best strategy would be to work throughout the life course, to bring people to the threshold of older age in good health, without any NCD.

Importance of an approach to risk reduction which challenges myths and stigma

The word 'dementia' originates from the Latin *demens*, which translates as 'no mind'. Colloquially, various pejorative terms for dementia have been used, including 'crazy', 'insane' and 'old-age stupor'.

In an attempt to reduce stigmatisation, the Japanese government decided in 2004 to change '*Chihō*', the Japanese word for dementia, to a less negative term '*Ninchishō*', meaning 'disease of cognition'. A year later, to embed the name change and raise awareness and understanding of dementia, the Japanese government subsidised a '10-year nationwide campaign to understand dementia and create dementia-friendly communities'.[21]

Some people have also objected to the use of the terms 'dementia' and 'Alzheimer's disease' in favour of more descriptive terms, such as 'memory loss' or 'forgetfulness'. However, some individuals with dementia wish to receive a specific diagnosis, as the diagnosis might finally make sense of a long period of not knowing what the root cause of particular symptoms was. Nonetheless, a person newly diagnosed with dementia should never be given that diagnosis alone without post-diagnostic support mechanisms.

Public understanding of dementia risk reduction is currently very low. There are several reasons for this:

1. The stigma of dementia and mental illness generally does not foster engagement.

2. The evidence supporting the case that behavioural or environmental modification will reduce dementia risk on an individual basis has been perceived as too weak to support widespread public information dissemination or other behaviour-change mechanisms.

3. Population-level evidence has by definition largely been derived from the commonest causes of dementia, namely sporadic Alzheimer's disease and vascular dementia.

In his seminal work, Goffman used the term 'stigma' to refer to 'an attribute that is deeply discrediting within a social interaction'. Individuals possessing such an attribute are different from others in ways that are undesired and shameful. The stigmatised individual is 'reduced…from a whole and usual person to a tainted, discounted one'.[22]

Stigmas are typically the attributes that, when observed by a majority group member, may lead to labelling, stereotyping, separation, status loss and discrimination.

Labelling and stereotyping involve the recognition of differences and the assignment of social salience to those differences. In the context of illness, labelling is the recognition that a person with a particular diagnosis differs from the norm in ways that have social significance.

Stereotyping is the assignment of negative attributions to these socially salient differences (i.e. the perception that the differences are undesirable).

In addition to public stigma, people with certain diagnostic labels may also experience self-stigma, or an 'internalisation' of the negative stereotypes held by the general public. This internalised or self-stigma may deter individuals from seeking treatment and social services, even when the opportunities are available, simply to avoid the stigma associated with that label.

Stigma can stop people living with dementia from engaging with risk-reduction initiatives. Communications on reducing dementia risk should be fully aligned with those on living well with dementia, ensuring that the public receive balanced messages that enable them to respond and plan appropriately.

Engagement with policy makers is needed to highlight the potential of dementia risk reduction and to support tailored approaches to public messaging. This in turn will help to make the case for greater research investment to enrich the evidence base.

The research and wider dementia community needs to highlight the importance of participating in research and raise awareness of initiatives such as *Join Dementia Research* that encourage public participation in research.[23]

The need to monitor, evaluate and improve the effectiveness of health promotion activities

In order to fill the research gap in health promotion and to answer the increasingly pertinent question of whether or not health promotion is a good investment, the World Health Organization commissioned a working group in 1995 to provide guidance on the appropriate methods for health promotion evaluation to increase their quality.

In England, thereafter, the Health Education Agency reviewed their experience of commissioning reviews of effectiveness and created a broader national platform for developing the evidence base for public health, subsequently developed by the Health Development Agency.

Health promotion initiatives should be evaluated in terms of their processes as well as their outcomes.

Adequate resources should be devoted to the evaluation of health promotion initiatives. Expertise in the evaluation of health promotion initiatives needs to be developed and sustained. Possible principles for the evaluation of health promotion initiatives include those listed in Box 3.5.

BOX 3.5 RESOURCE ALLOCATION IN HEALTH PROMOTION ACTIVITIES

Participation – at each stage of evaluation those with an interest should be involved.

Multiple methods – evaluations should draw on a variety of disciplines and employ a broad range of research methods.

Capacity building – evaluations should enhance the capacity of individuals, communities and organisations.

Appropriateness – evaluations should be designed to accommodate the complex nature of health promotion interventions and their long-term impact.

Notes

1. Forster, K. (2017) 'Third of dementia cases care preventable through nine lifestyle changes, say researchers.' Independent, 19 July 2017. Accessed on 2 October at www.independent.co.uk/news/health/dementia-cases-preventable-third-education-hearing-loss-lancet-university-college-london-a7849561.html

2. Alzheimer's Research UK (2015) 'Defeat dementia: The evidence and a vision for action.' Accessed on 6 November 2017 at www.alzheimersresearchuk.org/wp-content/uploads/2015/01/Defeat-Dementia-policy-report.pdf

3. Satizabal, C.L., Beiser, A.S., Chouraki, V., Chêne, G., Dufouil, C. and Seshadri, S. (2016) 'Incidence of dementia over three decades in the Framingham Heart Study.' New England Journal of Medicine 374, 6, 523–532. Accessed on 2 October 2017 at www.nejm.org/doi/full/10.1056/NEJMoa1504327

4. NHS Choices, 'Vascular dementia.' Accessed on 2 October 2017 at www.nhs.uk/Conditions/vascular-dementia/Pages/Introduction.aspx

5. Mitchell, S., Ridley, S.H., Sancho, R.M. and Norton M. (2016) 'The future of dementia risk reduction research: Barriers and solutions.' *Journal of Public Health*. Accessed on 2 October 2017 at https://doi.org/10.1093/pubmed/fdw103

6. Smith, B.J., Ali, S. and Quach, H. (2014) 'Public knowledge and beliefs about dementia risk: A national survey of Australians.' *BMC Public Health 14*, 661. Accessed on 2 October 2017 at www.ncbi.nlm.nih.gov/pmc/articles/PMC4226999

7. Accessed on 2 October 2017 at https://en.oxforddictionaries.com/definition/evidence

8. www.dementiasplatform.uk

9. www.neurodegenerationresearch.eu

10. NICE guideline [NG16] (2015). Accessed on 1 September 2017 at www.nice.org.uk/guidance/ng16

11. Norton, S., Matthews, F.E., Barnes, D.E., Yaffe, K. and Brayne, C. (2014) 'Potential for primary prevention of Alzheimer's disease: An analysis of population-based data.' *The Lancet Neurology 13*, 8, 788–794.

12. Cracknell, K. (2017) 'Interview: Sir Muir Gray on his plans for preventive healthcare.' *Health Club Management*, issue 5. Accessed on 2 October 2017 at www.healthclubmanagement.co.uk/health-club-management-features/Interview-Sir-Muir-Gray-on-his-plans-for-preventative-healthcare/31819

13. Valenzuela, M.J. and Sachdev, P. (2006) 'Brain reserve and cognitive decline: A non-parametric systematic review.' *Psychological Medicine 36*, 8, 1065–1073.

14. World Health Organization, The Ottawa Charter for Health Promotion. Accessed on 1 September 2017 at www.who.int/healthpromotion/conferences/previous/ottawa/en

15. Accessed on 1 September 2017 at http://nhfshare.heartforum.org.uk/RMAssets/Reports/Blackfriars%20consensus%20%20_V18.pdf

16. Accessed on 1 September 2017 at www.healthcheck.nhs.uk

17. Chief Medical Officer's Report 2011, 'Risk factors.' Accessed on 2 October 2017 at www.ssehsactive.org.uk/userfiles/Documents/rsikfactors.pdf

18. Accessed on 1 September 2017 at http://fingertips.phe.org.uk/profile-group/mental-health/profile/dementia

19. Accessed on 2 October 2017 at www.nice.org.uk/guidance/ng16

20. Soames Job, R.F. (1988) 'Effective and ineffective use of fear in health promotion campaigns.' *Am J Public Health* 78, 2, 163–167. Accessed on 7 November 2017 at www.ncbi.nlm.nih.gov/pmc/articles/PMC1349109

21. Hayashi, M. (2017) 'The Dementia Friends initiative – supporting people with dementia and their carers: reflections from Japan.' *International Journal of Care and Caring 1*, 2, 281–287. Accessed on 2 October at www.ingentaconnect.com/contentone/tpp/ijcc/2017/00000001/00000002/art00009

22. Goffman, E. (1963) *Stigma*. London: Penguin, p.3.

23. www.joindementiaresearch.nihr.ac.uk

4

Person-centred dementia care

This chapter is about person-centred care (PCC), a huge area – and one which is absolutely fundamental.

It's possible not to be very person-centred by using highly stigmatising labels such as 'demented', 'crazy' or 'mad'.

'Person-centredness' is a term that is becoming increasingly familiar within health and social care at a global level. It is being used to describe a standard of care that ensures that the patient is at the centre of care delivery.

Person-centred nursing was developed by McCormack and McCance, building on the work of Carl Rogers among others.[1] It is an approach to practice that focuses on how healthcare providers relate to people in need of care, others significant to the lives of these people and colleagues and other care providers. A definition is provided thus:

> [Person-centredness is] an approach to practice established through the formation and fostering of healthful relationships between all care providers, service users and others significant to them in their lives. It is underpinned by values of respect for persons (personhood), individual right to self-determination, mutual respect and understanding. It is enabled by cultures of empowerment that foster continuous approaches to practice development.[2]

It is not surprising that the body of literature relating to person-centred care is growing, along with the academic debate and critical dialogue regarding the development of this concept.

71

Person-centredness is not a new concept, but its exact roots in relation to 'humanistic psychology' continue to attract scrutiny.

Person-centredness reflects the concept of 'caring', and is underpinned by values of mutual respect, understanding for persons and individual right to self-determination. McCormack, in his original research, identifies mutuality in the therapeutic relationship as central to the process of shared decision-making, which recognises others' values as being of equal importance in decision-making.[3]

Some principles have been proposed.

BOX 4.1 SOME PRINCIPLES AND FEATURES OF PERSON-CENTRED APPROACHES

Four key principles of person-centred care

Principle 1. Being person-centred means affording people dignity, respect and compassion.

Principle 2. Being person-centred means offering coordinated care, support or treatment.

Principle 3. Being person-centred means offering personalised care, support or treatment.

Principle 4. Being person-centred means being enabling.[4]

But some care is needed here. Dewing and McCormack warn that:

It is here where the definitions being proposed in a number of influential policy documents are a particular cause for concern – they encourage many local policy-makers and healthcare managers to believe that person-centredness can be implemented and measured in a technical and concrete way and that the time needed to achieve and 'tick off' the introduction of person-centredness is much less than we know is really needed to achieve a transformed culture.[5]

It is pivotal not to get the term 'person-centred' mixed up with the term 'patient-centred'. The term 'patient-centred' is used frequently in several jurisdictions including the UK, the USA and Australia. Although this is linked to the individualised care element of person-centred care, it provides a much narrower focus than person-centred care, in that the person can only express those individual needs that are within their role as a patient.

Care partners are often torn between protecting the person with dementia and promoting his or her independence. Individuals with dementia and their family and friends, in reality, often struggle to preserve a 'pre-dementia self', while at the same time accommodating the diagnosis and assimilating the biological condition into a new identity.

The following aspects may be especially important.

- A person-centred healthcare system is one that supports people to make informed decisions about and successfully manage their own health and care.

- Person-centred care focuses on the individual needs of a person rather than on efficiencies of the care provider; builds upon the strengths of a person; and honours their values, choices and preferences.

- A person-centred model of care reorients the medical disease-dominated model of care that can be impersonal to those oriented to holistic wellbeing that encompasses all four human dimensions: bio–psycho–social–spiritual.

There is now a growing momentum behind human rights-based approaches and, with acknowledgement that dementia is a disability, an increasing awareness of the rights of people with dementia enshrined in the UN Convention on Rights of Persons with Disabilities.

VIPS framework

Dawn Brooker, in her contribution, acknowledges that person-centred care is not easy to describe in a straightforward manner.

In the VIPS framework, Brooker summarises Kitwood's philosophy of PCC for persons with dementia into four major elements with the acronym 'VIPS'.[6] The original VIPS definition was a reaction to policy definitions in the UK at that time which were interpreting person-centred care simply as individualised care. The VIPS definition was an attempt to spell out the different threads of person-centred care, while maintaining the sophistication of Tom Kitwood's original vision.[7]

The framework is outlined in Box 4.2.

BOX 4.2 VIPS FRAMEWORK

V (**Va**luing people): A value base that asserts the absolute value of all human lives, regardless of age or cognitive ability

I (**I**ndividualised care): An individualised approach, recognising uniqueness

P (**P**ersonal perspectives): Understanding the world from the perspective of the person identified as needing support

S (**S**ocial environment): Providing a social environment that supports psychological needs

---

The four features outlined in Box 4.2 are crucial for creating and sustaining a positive care culture in an organisation, which will help to develop and maintain frontline action that promotes positive care experiences for people living with dementia and other complex needs.

Although it was originally designed with care homes in mind, it is intended that the concept and format of the VIPS toolkit could readily be adapted to meet the needs of a range of environments or organisations, as has already been done for domiciliary care services and day centres.

Person-centred care can provide insights into the experiences of the person with dementia and support care approaches and solutions to meet individual needs. The individual experience of dementia will be determined in part by the social environment. Much can be done to ensure that the social environment is generally supportive of the needs of people with dementia.

BOX 4.3 NATIONAL OCCUPATION STANDARDS ON UPHOLDING RIGHTS AND ADDRESSING NEEDS AND PREFERENCES OF INDIVIDUALS

National Occupational standard SCDHSC0234 – 'Upholding the rights of individuals' – identifies the individual's right to be in control of their lives, to be respected for who they are, and to have information about themselves kept private.

National Occupational Standard SCDHSC0414 – 'Assess individual preferences and needs' – identifies the requirements when you assess the preferences and the care or support needs of individuals. This begins by working with individuals to carry out a comprehensive assessment of their preferences, needs and strengths, and the outcomes they wish to achieve through care or support.

Needs and care plans

Needs can be various – for example, physical, emotional, social, spiritual, communication, support or care needs. Care partners are the first people that a service user meets when a health need has arisen and they act as gate-keepers for subsequent care. It is important to competently and efficiently take an initial history and assessment of the service user's condition to enable care to be planned and implemented speedily.

Care or support plans are an important source of information as these are dynamic records that are constantly reviewed and updated in response to changing needs and preferences. A review will look with the individual at what is working, what doesn't work and what might need to change. It is perhaps constructive to think of care plans as 'living documents'; individuals themselves, their family, visitors and staff all are free to contribute.

Properly maintained care plans should mean that workers changing shifts or returning from holidays and temporary or agency workers will always have up-to-date information on the individual, enabling them to provide the best possible person-centred care.

Admiral Nurses from Dementia UK are UK-based qualified mental health nurses who have specialised in dementia care. Admiral Nurses can also work with the care partner/care-recipient dyad to identify dementia care services appropriate to their needs. Admiral Nurses may continue to support care partners throughout the milestones of the illness, including end-of-life care and beyond, as they are required to meet their care needs too.

The role of family and care partners in person-centred care and support of people with dementia

Changes in dementia may affect the relationships and roles of people with dementia, as close relatives (e.g. husband/wife, daughter/son, sister/brother) have to take on the role of informal care partner. These relatives' relationships with the person with dementia may change as a result of dementia, including challenges concerning 'Who am I?' and 'Who is she/he?'

Supporting a friend or relative with dementia is often highly stressful and can have a profound impact on the health and wellbeing of care partners.

Care partners often find themselves isolated. It is known that family care partners often look for continuity of care and flexibility; information about aids and entitlements; ongoing opportunities to talk to supportive professionals; specialist support; signposting to appropriate statutory and voluntary services; individually tailored information; peer support.

'Care partner stress' is usually defined as a multidimensional bio-psychosocial reaction resulting from an imbalance of care demands relative to care partners' personal time, social roles, physical and emotional states, financial resources and formal care resources, given the other multiple roles they fulfil.

To be fair, the act of caring can be an incredibly rewarding, loving, nurturing and fulfilling role as well as quite demanding. The term 'carer stress' ('caregiver burden' in some jurisdictions) may not capture linguistically the plethora of emotions that a care partner of an individual with dementia might experience. (Note: some people believe that the word 'care partner' itself is inadequate, reflected in the fact that many carers do not initially identify themselves with the role, at least initially.)

Language matters. As Brooker and Latham point out:

> Think about the type of language we commonly hear about dementia: 'time bomb', 'epidemic', 'burden', 'suffering'. Now imagine that you or someone close to you has just received a diagnosis of dementia. What images and underlying messages do those words send to you? Do they make you feel optimistic, hopeful, like there may be a light at the end of the tunnel? Or do they make you feel dispirited, demotivated, and overwhelmed? How might those feelings influence the way we think and behave towards people we encounter?[8]

There has been articulated a need to consider the reframing of the language of dementia care, and a need for the recognition of the diagnosed person's agency in the conduct of their day-to-day lives.[9]

Research has indicated that caregiving over a long period can have a negative impact on care partners, both mentally and physically. Given the magnitude of services provided and the sacrifices made by care partners, care partner stress has been recognised as a serious public health concern.

Numerous studies have reported that caring for a person with dementia is more stressful than caring for a person with a physical disability.

Predictors of care partner stress in dementia have also been well studied. Studies have shown that being a woman, providing care to a spouse, lower income status and the presence of significant behavioural problems in the patient are the most consistent factors associated with higher strain among care partners. However, interventions have been found to reduce care partners' stress and depression levels, improve care partners' quality of life and delay patients' nursing home placement.[10]

Care partner stress can increase the risk of depression and anxiety disorder, and informal care partners of people with dementia living at home experience care as more burdensome compared with informal care partners of recently institutionalised people with dementia.

How a person-centred approach can be implemented, including the use of advance planning and life story work

Advance care planning (ACP) is a 'process of discussion that usually takes place in anticipation of a future deterioration of a person's condition, between that person and a care worker'[11] usually from a healthcare background.

Developed largely in the United States, Australia and Canada, ACP is a process of communication that involves people in decisions about future care, making plans to ensure their preferences can be met when their mental capacity is lost.

Advance care planning includes wishes regarding care and treatment in the later stages of dementia, including preferred place of death and whether the patient wishes to discuss an advance care plan for end-of-life issues.

In England and Wales, it is recognised that, under common law, a specific anticipatory statement (usually advance refusal of medical treatment) has legal status. The Mental Capacity Act 2005 seeks to ensure that people without mental capacity are enabled to make their wishes and preferences for care and support known, so that these will be carried out.

A person's needs may change as the disease progresses

Talking about the 'severity' of dementia is sometimes not altogether helpful in that the progression of dementia is very often not linear and predictable.

However, possibly, some broad categories might be made (see Box 4.4). These are pretty 'rough and ready' and very approximate. We all change – but the point is that here care needs substantially change as the dementia advances.

BOX 4.4 BROAD DESCRIPTIONS OF 'MILD', 'MODERATE' AND 'SEVERE' DEMENTIA

Mild dementia

People experiencing mild dementia may still be able to function independently. However, they will experience memory lapses that can affect daily life, such as forgetting words or where things are.

Moderate dementia

People experiencing moderate dementia will likely need more assistance in their daily lives. It becomes harder to independently perform regular daily activities and self-care as dementia progresses.

Severe dementia

People will experience, in severe dementia, further mental decline as well as worsening physical capabilities and rapidly increasing needs and dependence.

How to adapt the physical environment to meet the changing needs of people with dementia

Most people with dementia wish to remain in their own homes for as long as possible, but as a person's dementia progresses they may find everyday tasks more difficult. These can range from using the stairs to taking medication. It is worth noting that people with dementia often find it comforting to have access to 'familiar possessions' in their immediate environment.

Using equipment and making adaptations to the home environment can help someone to continue to do things for themselves for longer. This can help the person with dementia to stay independent, and can offer family and care partners the reassurance of the person's safety and security.

Thus, an important goal in health promotion is to create home environments that support healthy ageing. Design of the physical environment is increasingly recognised as an important aid in the care of people with dementia. Facility administrators and designers now view the design of long-term care, assisted living and other environments as more than simply decorative.

In the ENABLE-AGE project (to examine the home environment and its importance for major components of healthy ageing), researchers used the term 'healthy ageing' to address selected aspects of physical, mental and social health that are assumed to be particularly relevant to housing.[12]

Among the core concepts chosen for the project were independence in daily activities and subjective wellbeing. It is widely accepted that an active life is positively associated with better health.

Engagement in 'meaningful activities' is of crucial importance in promoting and maintaining health and wellbeing throughout life, and thus independence in daily activities constitutes an important aspect of health in very old age.

Types of equipment designed to help older people with problems in general are often very useful for people with dementia

There are a range of different types of memory aids for helping people to remember the date, appointments, shopping lists and other things. These include noticeboards where people can write messages and reminders, and clocks with large faces that are easier to read.

Some people may have difficulty getting into and out of baths, or problems sitting down or standing up from the bottom of the bath tub. Transfer benches, grab rails or bath steps may be useful in this situation.

Some people with dementia may lose continence, which can be distressing and embarrassing. A multidisciplinary approach, perhaps involving a continence advisor and occupational therapist, can be helpful here.

The person's background, culture and experiences when providing their care

All too often, persons with dementia can become 'dehumanised' in the experience of receiving help from the NHS and social care.

In McCormack's formulation, four aspects of person-centred care are taken as a benchmark:

- being in relation (*social relationships*)

- being in a social world (*biography and relationships*)

- being in place (*environmental conditions*)

- being with self (*individual values*).[13]

Individuals with dementia and care partners tend to identify personal characteristics in frontline workers – for example, gender, ethnicity and cultural background – as important, in addition to personal qualities such as patience, compassion, sensitivity and empathy. Skills to help perform their role are also valued.

Historically, and still today, people living with dementia have been treated as if they are non-persons. Once people have the label of dementia, it is often assumed that they can no longer speak on their own behalf. This has been vigorously challenged in recent years. As dementia progresses, however, it can bring high levels of dependency.

It can become increasingly difficult to recognise the personhood behind the label. From one viewpoint, we should aspire to treat people with dementia at all stages of their disability in the way in which all people would wish to be treated. In Tom Kitwood's writing, the ethical standing of people with dementia was discussed in terms of personhood: 'Personhood…carries essentially ethical connotations: to be a person is to have a certain status, to be worthy of respect.'[14]

Dewing argues that Kitwood has indeed influenced the way in which person-centred practice is generally conceptualised in care services, but the significance of his definition is rarely critiqued.[15] In Dewing's striking contribution, it has been suggested that definitions of persons and personhood need to take account of the body and time, and gerontological nursing may want to reassess how much allegiance is given to basing nursing frameworks on the concept of personhood.

On a pragmatic level, the lack of status and value that is attached to people with dementia also sometimes extends to those who want to look after their family members with dementia and those whose employment involves caring.

The importance of clear documentation to communicate the care needs of the person with dementia from the interdisciplinary team

---

BOX 4.5 NATIONAL OCCUPATIONAL STANDARDS ON PLANNING CARE

National Occupational Standard CHS233 – 'Contribute to the assessment of needs and the planning, evaluation and review of individualised programmes of care for individuals' – covers working as a member of an interdisciplinary team through contributing to the assessment of service users' needs, contributing to the planning of individualised programmes of care, and contributing to evaluation and review.

The term 'interdisciplinary team' has been used to mean teams formed of practitioners drawn from different professions (or different disciplines within a profession) who are working together as a coordinated team to achieve agreed objectives with service users.

A care plan is a required document that sets out in detail the way daily care and support must be provided to an individual.

Personalised care and support planning encourages care professionals and people with long-term conditions and their care partners to work together to clarify and understand what is important to that individual.

Care plans agree goals, identify support needs, develop and implement action plans and monitor progress. This is a planned and continuous process, not a one-off event.

'I statements' from National Voices are about what matters to patients. Examples of 'I statements' to do with care planning are shown in Box 4.6.[16]

BOX 4.6 | STATEMENTS

I work with my team to agree a care and support plan.

I know what is in my care and support plan.

I know what to do if things change or go wrong.

I have as much control of planning my care and support as I want.

I can decide the kind of support I need and how to receive it.

I have regular, comprehensive reviews of my medicines.

I have systems in place to get help at an early stage to avoid a crisis.

Services need to work with individuals to discuss and record information in a way that is accessible to the patient, using language that is easily understood. This could involve the use of advocacy services, interpretation and translation services, peer support or the provision of information in alternative formats, such as easy-read, pictorial or audio.

Where individuals have a disability, impairment or sensory loss, NHS organisations are legally required to follow the Accessible Information Standard and provide information that can be easily read or understood and to support individuals in communicating with services.

Care planning should take place as soon as possible after diagnosis (irrespective of where that happens) and the frequency of reviews should be responsive to the needs of all individuals diagnosed with dementia.

Outcomes of a care plan are a key measure of its efficacy and assessing this is important.

NHS England argues that a dementia care plan should cover D.E.M.E.N.T.I.A.[17] (see Box 4.7).

BOX 4.7 'D.E.M.E.N.T.I.A.'

D: Diagnosis review

E: Effective support for care partners review

M: Medication review

E: Evaluate risk

N: New symptoms inquiry

T: Treatments and support

I: Individuality

A: Advance care planning

The value of person-centred care in therapeutic relationships and communication

Relationships are very important to all of us. Relationships in dementia care remain the overlooked variable in many studies, with very few having explored the dynamics between the parties involved.

McCormack proposes that relationships, environmental conditions and individual values epitomise person-centred gerontological nursing.[17]

A shift in thinking about what it is to care is happening.

Nolan and colleagues have developed and empirically tested the Senses Framework; they suggest that the person receiving care, family care partners and paid care partners should all experience relationships that promote 'the Senses'.[18] The fundamental premise is that good care which is relationship-centred can only be delivered when the Senses are experienced by all parties.[19]

There has been increasing interest in the notion of 'dementia care triads': the person with dementia, the care partner and the clinician. For example, it is possible that there might be two types of communication that can occur in this triad: 'enabling' dementia communication and 'disabling' dementia communication.

Communication is discussed further in Chapter 5.

In some instances, there is evidence that the care partners have plainly disregarded the views of the individual with dementia. This is clearly unacceptable.

Admiral Nurses do try to balance the perspectives of the individuals living with dementia and care partners; however, there are situations where conflicting situations can arise. These decisions seem to arise from a desire to enhance the welfare of both the people diagnosed with dementia and the care partners.

Care partners sometimes get frustrated because they are not involved in the decision-making; however, it is also possible that sometimes they just accepted these decisions. Researchers have found themselves faced with real dilemmas when deciding *whose* needs are more important. For instance, a care partner may want a break from caregiving but the care recipient cannot understand why s/he has to go into respite care.

The importance of person-centred approaches in the management and development of services

---

BOX 4.8 NATIONAL OCCUPATIONAL STANDARDS
ON LEADING SERVICE DELIVERY

National Occupational Standard SCDHSC0415 – 'Lead the service delivery planning process to achieve outcomes for individuals' – outlines the requirements for leading the service delivery planning process to achieve outcomes that will meet individuals' preferences and needs. It includes developing, agreeing, monitoring and reviewing service delivery plans for health, social or other care services. It also includes making any adjustments necessary to service delivery plans to improve outcomes for individuals.

The importance of flexibility, choice in services, control and personalised care to disabled people and older people has been consistently argued, and is a key feature in perceptions of high-quality services. Overcoming inflexibility in service provision is particularly important. It has been argued that choice for users improves the quality of care.

The provision of services for minority ethnic groups exemplifies the challenge of ensuring flexibility and responsiveness. Service users reported better experiences of care from specialised services, but a focus on specialist services may inadvertently stop mainstream services from improving.

Notes

1. McCormack, B. and McCance, T. (2010) *Person-Centred Nursing: Theory and Practice*. Chichester: Wiley-Blackwell.
2. McCormack, B. and McCance, T. (eds) (2017) *Person-Centred Practice in Nursing and Health Care*, 2nd edition. Oxford: Wiley-Blackwell, p.3.
3. McCormack, B. (2003) 'A conceptual framework for person-centred practice with older people.' *Int J Nurs Pract 9*, 3, 202–209.
4. Collins, A. (2014) *'Measuring wat really matters.'* Thought paper, April 2014, The Health Foundation. Accessed on 1 September 2017 at www.health.org.uk/sites/health/files/MeasuringWhatReallyMatters.pdf
5. Dewing, J. and McCormack, B. (2017) Editorial: 'Tell me, how do you define person-centredness?' *Journal of Clinical Nursing 17–18*, 2509–2510.
6. Brooker, D. and Latham, I. (2016) *Person-Centred Dementia Care: Making Services Better with the VIPS Framework*, 2nd edition. London: Jessica Kingsley Publishers.
7. Kitwood, T. (1997) *Dementia Reconsidered: The Person Comes First*. Buckingham: Open University Press.
8. Brooker, D. and Latham, I. (2016) *Person-Centred Dementia Care: Making Services Better with the VIPS Framework*, 2nd edition. London: Jessica Kingsley Publishers, p.57.

9. Sabat, S.R., Johnson, A., Swarbrick, C. and Keady, J. (2011) 'The "demented other" or simply "a person"? Extending the philosophical discourse of Naue and Kroll through the situated self.' *Nursing Philosophy 12*, 4, 282–292; discussion 293–296.

10. Andrén, S. and Elmståhl, S. (2007) 'Relationships between income, subjective health and caregiver burden in caregivers of people with dementia in group living care: a cross-sectional community-based study.' *Int J Nurs Stud 44*, 3, 435–446.

11. National Council for Palliative Care (2007) 'Advance Care Planning: A Guide for Health and Social Care Staff.' Accessed on 7 November 2017 at www.ncpc.org.uk/sites/default/files/AdvanceCarePlanning.pdf

12. Iwarsson, S., Wahl, H.W., Nygren, C., Oswald, F. *et al.* (2007) 'Importance of the home environment for healthy aging: Conceptual and methodological background of the European ENABLE-AGE Project.' *Gerontologist 47*, 1, 78–84.

13. McCormack, B. (2004) 'Person-centredness in gerontological nursing: an overview of the literature.' *J Clin Nurs 13*, 3a, 31–8.

14. Kitwood, T. and Bredin, K. (1992) 'Towards a theory of dementia care: personhood and well-being.' *Ageing and Society 12*, 269–287, 275.

15. Dewing, J. (2008) 'Personhood and dementia: Revisiting Tom Kitwood's ideas.' *International Journal of Older People Nursing 3*, 1, 3–13.

16. See, for example, the Publications page on the National Voices website, www.nationalvoices.org.uk/publications/our-publications/narrative-person-centred-coordinated-care

17. NHS England (2017) 'Dementia: Good care planning: Information for primary care providers and commissioners.' Accessed on 1 September 2017 at www.england.nhs.uk/wp-content/uploads/2017/02/dementia-good-care-planning.pdf

18. Nolan, M. R., Brown, J., Davies, S., Nolan, J. et al. (2006) 'The Senses Framework: improving care for older people through a relationship-centred approach.' *Getting Research into Practice (GRiP) Report No 2*. University of Sheffield.

19. Watson, J. (2016) 'Developing the Senses Framework to support relationship-centred care for people with advanced dementia until the end of life in care homes.' *Dementia (London)*, doi: 10.1177/1471301216682880

5

Communication, interaction and behaviour in dementia care

The importance of effective communication in dementia care

Communication is a complex process, which involves and requires many aspects of cognitive and social skills.

Communication is achieved through speech, writing, gesture, posture, gaze, affect/mood and intonation. These are specific to the place and purpose, or the context, of the communication. Care staff need to be aware of how residents signal the need to communicate and how to react to the signals.

If any degree of brain injury impairs any of these skills, then it can affect the ability to communicate successfully.

Communication refers to exchanges between individuals and social interactions. It occupies a central place in participation in social activities and can be severely impaired by conditions affecting the brain.

We tend to think of communication as only talking, but in fact it consists of much more than that. Much communication takes place through non-verbal communication such as gestures, facial expression and touch. Non-verbal communication is particularly important for a person with dementia who may be losing their language skills. When a person with dementia behaves in ways that cause problems for their care partner, they might be trying to communicate something.

BOX 5.1 NATIONAL OCCUPATIONAL STANDARDS ON COMMUNICATION

National Occupational Standard SFHGEN97 – 'Communicate effectively in a healthcare environment' – is about communicating effectively with individuals in a healthcare environment. You will be expected to communicate effectively with a number of people in a variety of situations.

National Occupational Standard SCDHSC0031 – 'Promote effective communication' – identifies the requirements when you promote effective communication within a work setting where individuals are cared for or supported.

Some important points:

- Use familiar words and phrases that you know will be understood in communicating with someone with a language disorder.

- Intensive questioning can be overwhelming.

- Tone of voice can convey different feelings.

- Finally, *don't rush*, as information can be lost if you speak too quickly.

The impact of memory and language difficulties on communication

Memory and language difficulties can have different effects on communication.

Memory difficulties

A person with memory problems may find it hard to access information that they 'know'.

This can affect skills such as word recall and remembering people's names, which are very important when communicating socially.

The failure to remember names or faces at a party, or information relevant to a conversation, can cause social embarrassment.

There are strategies and cues you can use to help the person with dementia better accomplish these activities, maintain some independence and control over the environment and reduce the need for him or her to repetitively ask for missing information.

These could include:

- the use of labels or pictures on cupboards to show content (e.g. coffee cup)

- prominently displaying clocks and calendars.

Language difficulties

Problems with language can occur in all forms of dementia.

This is because the diseases that cause dementia can affect the parts of the brain that generate and understand language. How and when language problems develop will depend on the individual, as well as the type of dementia and the stage it is at.

These problems might also vary from day to day. In some forms of dementia – such as frontotemporal dementia – it is very likely to be one of the first symptoms that is noticed.

One sign that a person's language is being affected by dementia is that they can't find the right words. They may use a related or similar word (e.g. 'book' for 'newspaper'), use substitutes for words (e.g. 'thing to sit on' instead of 'chair') or may not find any words at all.

Dementia can also affect the person's ability to make a socially appropriate response, which may or may not reflect problems in understanding or expressing language.

There may eventually come a time when the person can hardly communicate at all using language.

Checking that communication has been understood is an essential part of the process. A vital skill that checks understanding is summarising. A summary should bring together the main points of an exchange of information. This will allow the individual to correct you if necessary.

Social cognitive changes

A person with dementia, for example, quite early on with the behavioural variant of frontotemporal dementia, might show lack of empathy with others, behave in a certain way (e.g. impulsively or in a disinhibited, inappropriate way) or make 'faux pas' utterances. These are fundamentally different from memory or language problems, reflecting changes in a different underlying neuronal network.

Active listening skills

Active listening is the highest and most effective level of listening, and it is a special communication skill.

It is based on complete attention to what a person is saying, listening carefully while showing interest and not interrupting. Active listening requires listening for the content, intent and feeling of the speaker.

Active listening can help to improve communication between you and the person you're caring for. Active listening is very important (see Box 5.2).

BOX 5.2 ACTIVE LISTENING

- Use eye contact to look at the person, and encourage him or her to look at you when you are talking.
- Use touch (handshake, hand-holding).
- Try not to interrupt.
- Stop what you're doing so you can give the person your full attention while he or she speaks.
- Minimise all distractions.

Gaining a person's attention before asking a question or beginning a task with them

Social communication difficulties are particularly associated with injury to the frontal lobes of the brain.

Difficulties in this area can mean the person does not recognise everyday social cues, both verbal and non-verbal. For example, they may not realise that someone is uncomfortable with the topic of conversation or that they are in a hurry to leave.

The importance of speaking clearly, calmly and with patience
Speak clearly

Speak clearly, calmly and slowly to allow the person time to understand information. Use simple, short sentences and avoid direct questions. Keep choices to a minimum and don't raise your voice.

Body language

People with dementia may find it difficult to understand what is being said, but can be quick to interpret the message on people's faces and may still be aware of body language.

Smile warmly, make eye contact, make sure you are at the person's level and use a friendly tone.

Show respect and patience

Adapt what you are saying if the person with dementia does not understand. Don't rush.

Listen

Listen carefully to what the person has to say, giving plenty of encouragement, while looking out for other clues to what they might be trying to communicate.

Talk to the person

A person with dementia may find it difficult to understand or be slow at finding the right words.

Adaptation of the environment to minimise sensory difficulties experienced by an individual with dementia

A number of people with dementia will have some form of sensory impairment (such as sight loss, hearing loss or both).

People with both sensory impairments and dementia are likely to have additional difficulties with their communication. However, there is still a lot you can do to help them communicate effectively.

Hearing loss

Both dementia and hearing loss can make people feel socially isolated, so having both conditions at once can be very difficult. This makes good communication extremely important.

Most people over 70 will have some degree of hearing loss. They may consider themselves to be deaf, 'hard of hearing' or having 'acquired hearing loss'. This may be due to age-related damage or other causes (such as noise damage, infection, disease or injury).

In comparison, people who are born deaf or become deaf at a young age are considered to have 'profound deafness'.

How a person with hearing loss communicates will depend on a range of factors including:

- the type of hearing loss they have

- whether they use a hearing aid, British Sign Language, lip-reading or a combination of all of them, personal preference and life history.

There are strong links between dementia and hearing loss, raising the possibility that hearing loss can make developing dementia more likely. This is research 'work in progress'.

Sight loss

Many people experience some degree of sight loss as they get older. It is estimated that 1.6 million people over 65 in the UK are living with sight loss.

This may be age-related possibly with identifiable definite aetiologies such as cataracts or macular degeneration. Many people with sight loss will need glasses to help them see.

People with sight loss are likely to experience more difficulties as a result of their dementia. Not being able to see what is around them can lead to a greater sense of disorientation and distress, as well as decreased mobility and a risk of falls.

Having both dementia and sight loss can also make people feel isolated from those around them. This makes good communication extremely important, and makes imperative the need to solve any reversible causes of sight impairment such as cataracts.

Communicating with a person with dementia and sight loss may be difficult as the person may not be able to pick up on non-verbal cues or follow a conversation as easily.

Adapting a home for a person with dementia requires changes to the physical space as well as changes to activities and the ways in which we interact with the person. In addition to the changes in vision or hearing that come with ageing, people with dementia often have more difficulty perceiving depth, discriminating between colours or seeing contrast.

Some changes to the home environment may help the person manage these difficulties.

The importance of ensuring that individuals have any required support (e.g. spectacles, hearing aids) to enable successful communication

Many patients may enter the hospital in a 'communication-vulnerable' state, or become so by virtue of their condition or treatment.

Possible solutions might include:

- a modified call bell (to help people who can't use a regular call bell to get help) and 'how to' instructions with easy-to-follow pictures

- a magnifying glass for people who don't have their glasses.

How life story information may enable or support more effective communication

In his seminal book *Dementia Reconsidered*,[1] Kitwood recognised these threats to the personhood of people with dementia and stated that biographical knowledge about a person 'becomes essential if that identity is still to be held in place'.

Kitwood and other authors subsequently have suggested that one way of holding identity in place is through the conduct, production and use of a life story.

For people with dementia, however, the connection between past and present life events can become fractured and the meaning of shared stories difficult to follow.

This is because the telling of a chronological life story becomes challenged as a result of cognitive impairment and the sustained, progressive and deleterious impact on the person's autobiographical and semantic memory functioning, as well as their communication skills.

Commonly reported benefits usually include enhanced wellbeing improvements in mood and some components of cognitive function; and reductions in disorientation and anxiety and improvements in self-esteem, memory and social interaction.

The utility of a personal biography to contextualise and understand ageing has a relatively long history in the literature and in the 'hands-on' care of older people.

It is important for the listener to attempt to understand why the person is sharing that particular story, at that particular time, and then attempt to unpack its meaning from within the person's life course.

Locating and articulating a biographical connection between past and present life events is one way of preserving the narrator's personal identity and affirming a sense of agency and self. It is critical to continuity.

Adaptation of communication techniques according to the different abilities and preferences of people with dementia

Approaches or interventions that show promise but have not been empirically tested to assess impact on patient outcomes include those which aim to improve communication between clinical staff and the care partner.

You should try to do what you can to reduce any barriers to communication (see Boxes 5.3 and 5.4).

The most effective way to make sure that you are meeting someone's communication needs and providing person-centred care is to know as much as possible as you can about them.

A communication passport might be used by some which provides vital information about needs, wishes and preferences. These pull together the information into a format that is easy to read, often with pictures and photographs.

BOX 5.3 NATIONAL OCCUPATION STANDARDS ON SUPPORTING INDIVIDUALS WITH COMMUNICATION NEEDS

National Occupational Standard SCDHSC0369 – 'Support individuals with specific communication needs' – identifies the requirements when you support individuals who have specific communication needs. This includes identifying individuals' specific communication preferences and needs, supporting individuals to interact with other people and monitoring communication to identify changing needs.

BOX 5.4 EXAMPLES OF COMMUNICATION INTERVENTIONS

Braille and Braille software

Braille is a writing system which enables blind and partially sighted people to read and write through touch. It consists of patterns of raised dots arranged in cells of up to six dots in a 3 x 2 configuration. Each cell represents a letter, numeral or punctuation mark.

British Sign Language

British Sign Language is a method of non-verbal communication that uses movements of the hands, body, face and head, which make up a complete language system. It is the preferred first language of many deaf people and is used by hearing people to communicate with those who are deaf.

Technological aids

Hearing aids, hearing loops, text phones, text messaging on mobile phones and magnifiers are all forms of technological communication devices.

Advocate

This is a nominated person who will act or speak on behalf of other individuals who may not be able to put forward their opinions due to communication difficulties.

Talking Mats

'Talking Mats' consist of a textured mat on which picture symbols are placed as a conversation progresses.

How behaviours seen in people with dementia may be a means for communicating unmet needs

Behaviour is communication. Whether it's good, bad or indifferent, it is a clear expression of our feelings and needs.

People with dementia frequently lose the ability to speak as the disease progresses. However, they continue to communicate in other ways – through body language, gestures and facial expressions.

How a person's feelings and perception may affect their behaviour

We communicate mainly through facial expressions, body language, gestures and touch.

Non-verbal communication is important, and provides clues about how someone is feeling and what they are trying to communicate (see Box 5.5).

BOX 5.5 OVERVIEW OF NON-VERBAL COMMUNICATION

Eye contact

Eye contact is essential when communicating as it lets the receiver know you are listening, showing an interest and understanding messages.

Facial expressions

Facial expressions tell us what people are thinking even when they do not realise it. Sometimes, what we say is contradicted by what our body language is saying.

Gestures

Gestures are signals used with our body to convey messages. Gestures can be seen a lot when heated discussions are taking place and the message is important.

The behaviour of others might affect a person with dementia

How other people communicate can have an impact on the ability of the person with dementia to communicate.

- Slow up the interaction.

- Be patient and wait for a response.

- Maintain a comfortable and pleasant intonation pattern and non-linguistic communicative style via eye contact, smiles and a relaxed state.

Common causes of distressed behaviour by people with dementia

There are often good reasons why someone with dementia is distressed or behaving unusually. However, they might not always be able to tell you what's troubling them.

The challenge is to work out what the cause is and what you can do to help, for the benefit of both of you.

Sometimes we react to unusual behaviour without knowing what the person might need or be saying through their behaviour.

Others have used 'Stop' and 'Pause' to describe the key ways to help you listen and watch, in order to understand distressed and unusual behaviour.[2]

BOX 5.6 'STOP' AND 'PAUSE'

Stop

S – See things from the point of view of person with dementia

T – Think about your own thoughts and feelings

O – Observe and ask what the person is trying to communicate and what is going on

P – Patience and persistence

Pause

P – Physical

A – Activities

U – You

S – Self-esteem

E – Emotions

Recognition of distressed behaviour and responses to comfort or reassure the person with dementia

It is important to understand that distressed behaviours are not always due to dementia.

People with dementia show distressed patterns of behaviour for a reason, but they may be unable to explain this.

Check whether they are thirsty, hungry, too hot, too cold, in pain, need the toilet or are constipated. Check how they are feeling. Are they anxious? Have they forgotten they are in hospital and are trying to find the way home? Are they feeling unwell? Sometimes distressed behaviour is the only sign of an underlying physical illness such as an infection.

Due to illness or the stress of hospitalisation, people with dementia can be pushed beyond their limit of coping, become distressed and behave in ways that demonstrate they are disturbed.

Persons with dementia may become distressed or anxious and often, staff and care partners will not know why this happens or how to prevent and alleviate this distress. Distressed behaviours could be shouting, screaming, verbally aggressive comments or physical aggression.

A person's surroundings can also have an impact (e.g. if a person with dementia does not recognise their reflection in a mirror, they may become anxious that another person is in the room).

For ways in which you can help, see Box 5.7.

BOX 5.7 WAYS TO HELP IN SITUATIONS OF 'DISTRESSED BEHAVIOUR'

- Listen in a calm, affectionate and reassuring manner.
- Use verbal and non-verbal ways of reassuring.
- Avoid confrontation.
- Try to understand and meet the person's needs.
- Knowledge of the person and their history will help.
- Offer the person gentle reassurance.
- The person should have their eyesight and hearing tested, and if necessary should wear glasses and a hearing aid.

The notion that personhood can be maintained or diminished within relationships and social contexts is clearly exemplified through Kitwood's notion of malignant social psychology which surrounds dementia. That is, through stigmatisation of those around them individuals with dementia (IWD) can often be disempowered, infantilised, depersonalised and devalued through a predominant focus on negativity, deficit and disability.

The development of practices and services that meet the communication needs of people with dementia

The VERA framework has been developed specifically for health professionals working with people who have dementia. It provides a practical approach to achieving better communication.[3]

This useful tool describes a stage-by-stage process of communication that helps professionals to respond in a sensitive and compassionate manner. A primary idea that underpins VERA is that a person 'cannot not communicate'. Communication that is often labelled as 'impaired' can be meaningful if it is viewed as the actions of one person trying to connect with another. Communication shares a need, concern or experience.

Notes

1. Kitwood, T. (1997) *Dementia Reconsidered: The Person Comes First.* Buckingham: Open University Press, p.56.
2. Sussex Partnerships NHS Foundation Trust (2015) 'Helping someone with dementia who is distressed or behaving unusually – version 2.' Accessed on 1 September 2017 at www.sussexpartnership.nhs.uk/sites/default/files/documents/dementia_information_for_care partners_of_people_living_with_dementia_who_are_distressed_or_behaving_unusually_-_ver_2_-_oct_15.pdf
3. Blackhall, A., Hawkes, D., Hingley, D. and Wood S. (2011) 'VERA framework: Communicating with people who have dementia.' *Nursing Standard 26*, 10, 35–39.

6

Health and wellbeing in dementia care

It is important for individuals with dementia to maintain good physical and mental health through nutrition, exercise and a healthy lifestyle that includes social engagement.

Research has suggested that combining good nutrition with mental, social and physical activities may have a greater benefit in maintaining or improving brain health and neuroplasticity than any single activity.

Such intervention is particularly crucial from middle age onwards, when the brain faces a series of challenges that can include the pathogenesis of neurodegenerative diseases such as Alzheimer's disease.

Several molecular systems could potentially participate in the benefits of exercise on the brain.

It could be that being married is associated with a reduced risk of dementia compared to being widowed or lifelong single. This frames social engagement and social health as modifiable risk factors in prevention.[1] A number of studies show that more engagement in leisure activities is related to reduced risk of dementia or Alzheimer's disease.[2]

Anticipating an individual's health needs

Dementia is fast becoming one of the most pressing challenges for the care of older people, and the main contributor to disability and dependence. A critical aspect is to anticipate and prevent fatigue, a risk of falling, and problems in nutrition and hydration.

Fatigue

Daytime somnolence is commonly reported in patients with dementia with Lewy bodies (DLB), and it is a major stressor for care partners.

When daytime sleepiness is subjectively and objectively found in Alzheimer's disease, it is typically related to greater dementia severity.

Moreover, sleep fragmentation due to respiratory and movement-related arousal can occur in diffuse Lewy body dementia and Parkinson's disease, but it is not known if these episodes of nocturnal arousal are sufficient to interfere with daytime alertness.

For those who fall, the risk of sustaining a fracture is three times higher than for cognitively well people.[3] Also, those who fall are five times more likely to be hospitalised or live in a long-term care setting than older adults with dementia who do not fall. People with Parkinson's disease, vascular and Lewy body dementia are more prone to mobility disturbances.

Risk of falling

The person with dementia may experience changes that increase their risk of falling.

Changes may occur in:

- recognition of sensory input, such as sight, sound, touch

- coordination of movement between the brain and body

- interpretation of their environment, causing illusions and misperceptions

- initiation of mobility (particularly if living with concomitant frailty).

Things to consider when a person falls:

- Is there a reversible cause or is it related to another medical condition? Is the person taking multiple medications? Is the person experiencing medication side effects or interactions? Are medications being taken as prescribed?

- Does the person have changes in their vision?

- Has the person's mobility changed?

- Is the person in pain but unable to recognise or communicate their discomfort?

- Has the person developed a 'fear of falling' and what can you do to improve his or her confidence?

How the care partner communicates with the person they are assisting is an important factor in reducing the risk of falls for people with dementia.

Nutrition and hydration

Nutrition and hydration are essential to health and wellbeing. When well managed, they provide a vital contribution for people recovering from illness and for those at risk of malnutrition.

When managed poorly, they pose a significant threat to patient safety. Risks for, and prevalence of, malnutrition and dehydration are high in older people but even higher in older people with dementia.

Providing for nutrition and hydration must be carried out in a person-centred way. Efforts must be made to meet each individual's needs and choices. Their care plan is an essential part of recording and delivering this.

Interventions to support older people around eating and drinking vary: changing the size and colour of a plate, increasing exercise, altering the noise in the ambient environment or changing knowledge or attitudes; the full range of interventions may be helpful for people with dementia.

Important factors include social interactions of residents at mealtime; self-feeding ability; the dining environment; the attitudes, knowledge and skills of staff; adequate time to eat/availability of staff to provide assistance; sensory properties of the food; hospitality and mealtime logistics; choice and variety in the dining experience; and nutrient density of food.

Some National Occupation Standards are important (see Box 6.1).

BOX 6.1 NATIONAL OCCUPATIONAL STANDARDS ON FOOD AND DRINK

National Occupational Standard SCDHSC0213 – 'Provide food and drink to promote individuals' health and well-being' – identifies requirements when you provide food and drink for individuals who need support to eat and drink. This includes supporting individuals to communicate what they wish to eat and drink and preparing their selected food and drink.

National Occupational Standard SCDHSC0214 – 'Support individuals to eat and drink' – identifies the requirements when you support individuals who require assistance to consume food and drink.

National Occupational Standard SFHCHS68 – 'Support individuals with long term conditions to manage their nutrition' – This will involve reviewing relevant information about the individual's condition and confirming with them the actions being taken to manage their nutrition.

Signs and symptoms of poor nutrition and hydration

Nutritional problems, loss of appetite and weight loss are common problems in dementia, especially as the severity of illness increases.

Swallowing problems (dysphagia) become increasingly noticeable as dementia worsens.

Swallowing difficulties could be related to dementia, stroke, abscesses, tumours or degenerative neuromuscular diseases. Advice may be needed on management, options including using food thickeners with appropriate posture and feeding techniques.

Some features of poor nutrition are:

- feeling tired all the time

- increased infections

- constipation

- depression.

Some features of poor hydration:

- feelings of thirst as the body tries to increase fluid levels

- dark-coloured urine as the body tries to reduce fluid loss

- headaches, tiredness and confusion as the flow of blood to the brain decreases

- urinary tract infections, which are prevalent in some groups in care.

Unless their fluid intake is deliberately restricted for medical reasons, individuals should be encouraged to drink throughout the day and not wait until they feel thirsty, as feelings of thirst are an early sign of dehydration.

To make sure that individuals are drinking enough, you need to offer drinks and encourage and support them to drink as set out in their care plan.

Drinks need to be refreshed regularly and placed within easy reach for those with restricted movement or mobility.

If you are at all concerned about an individual's fluid intake, make sure you report these concerns to either a senior member of staff, the individual's care partner or their family.

Hunger

There are lots of ways to increase a person's appetite and interest in food and drink. Knowing the person will help, as everyone has their own routines, preferences and needs. You will also have a better idea about their likes and dislikes.

It's also important to think about what they can physically manage. Here are some ideas that may help:

- Make food look and smell appealing. Use different tastes, colours and smells. The aroma of cooking – for example, freshly baked bread – can stimulate someone's appetite.

- Look for opportunities to encourage the person to eat.

- Give the person food they actually like. Try not to overload the plate with too much food – small and regular portions often work best.

- Try different types of food or drinks. 'Favourite' foods or drinks can change.

- If food goes cold, it will lose its appeal. Consider serving half portions to keep food warm. Use a plate warmer or a microwave to reheat food.

How to recognise and manage pain in people with dementia

BOX 6.2 NATIONAL OCCUPATIONAL STANDARDS ON PHYSICAL COMFORT NEEDS

National Occupational Standard SCDHSC0216 – 'Help address the physical comfort needs of individuals' – identifies the requirements when you help address individuals' needs in relation to physical comfort. This includes assisting individuals to minimise the pain and discomfort they experience and helping to provide conditions that are suitable for individuals to rest.

People with dementia experience physical and psychological pain but, particularly if the dementia is advanced, may not be able to express this in conventional ways. It is important to identify appropriate terminology for individuals. For example, do they describe aching or discomfort?

It is also important to recognise non-verbal ways in which people might express pain – for example, through grimacing, flinching or guarding the painful area, restlessness or aggressive behaviour or pulling at tubes.

Today, there is extensive ongoing work to develop and test appropriate pain assessment instruments for people with advanced dementia. Most of the instruments are based on the assumption and recommendations of the American Geriatrics Society Panel that pain can be expressed by changes in facial expression (e.g. frowning), vocalisation and verbalisation (e.g. groaning) and body movements.[4]

If pain in a person with dementia goes unrecognised and untreated, there is a danger not only of the person suffering needlessly but also of them being prescribed inappropriate treatments for their changed behaviour. For example, if a person becomes withdrawn or distressed because of pain, they may be assumed to be depressed and prescribed antidepressants. Indeed, chronic pain can make a person depressed, but treating the underlying pain effectively should relieve both the pain and the depression.

If a person becomes aggressive or agitated because of pain, they may be prescribed inappropriate medications which potentially have serious side effects. Again, treating the underlying pain should alleviate the resulting problem behaviours.

Persistent pain can lead to decreased mobility.

The needs of people with dementia at the end of life may be different from those with different diseases.

Pain research in dying people with dementia is of particular interest for several reasons.

1. Research including elderly patients often excludes people with dementia and, until now, especially dying people with dementia.

2. Palliative care for cancer patients cannot necessarily be transferred to dying people with dementia.

3. The nature of dementia leads to reduction of the neurotransmitter acetylcholine, responsible for neuromuscular transmission, and the autonomic, sympathetic and parasympathetic nervous systems. Consequently, drugs that affect the cholinergic systems (anticholinergic drugs) potentially might have very dangerous effects.

Supporting an individual in maintaining personal appearance and hygiene

---

BOX 6.3 NATIONAL OCCUPATIONAL STANDARDS ON PERSONAL HYGIENE AND APPEARANCE

National Occupational Standard SCDHSC0218 – 'Support individuals with their personal care needs' – includes supporting individuals to access and use toilet facilities, to maintain their personal hygiene and to manage their personal appearance. It includes a role for supporting rights, choices, wellbeing and active participation.

National Occupational Standard SFHGEN105 – 'Enable individuals to maintain their personal hygiene and appearance' – covers enabling individuals to maintain their personal hygiene and appearance where they are in need of such assistance for whatever reason.

A person's appearance is integral to their self-respect and older people need to receive appropriate levels of support to maintain the standards they have been used to.

Personal preferences should be respected, as well as choice in how support is provided – for example, allowing people to choose when and how to carry out personal care tasks, using their own toiletries, allowing them to choose what to wear and how to style their hair, and having clean, ironed clothes that fit are all ways of maintaining control and identity.

Particular care should be taken in residential settings to ensure that personal laundry is treated with respect and not mixed up or damaged.

It is important to support people to maintain their personal hygiene and appearance, and their living environment, to at least the standards that they want.

- Allow plenty of time for tasks – for example, with washing and dressing.

- When providing support with personal care, take the individual's lifestyle choices into consideration – respect their choice of dress and hairstyle, for example.

- Don't make assumptions about appropriate standards of hygiene for individuals.

- Check that the care plan states the time the person wishes to be bathed or showered and ensure this is observed as far as possible.

Cleanliness in hospitals is regularly found to be one of the top five issues for patients. Having a clean home is particularly important to older women in terms of maintaining their dignity and self-respect.

The NHS 'Essence of Care' benchmark[5] for personal and oral hygiene focuses on assessment of need, planned care based on negotiation with patients, the care environment and appropriate levels of assistance.

There are things you can do to make the experience of washing and bathing less frightening and embarrassing, and safer for both parties:

- Ensure bathing is viewed as a relaxing experience.

- If the person doesn't like water in their face, use a damp facecloth or wipe to wash their face before/after a shower.

- Help the person feel independent by allowing them to be as involved as they want in bathing.

Some people find it easier to be bathed by someone they don't know, such as a care worker.

The impact of delirium, depression and social stressors

Dementia is very common in people admitted to acute hospitals, affecting one in four patients. Six per cent of people living with dementia are inpatients in acute hospitals at any given time.[6]

Dementia is often unrecognised by doctors and other hospital staff and frequently complicated by delirium. The type of dementia is also a factor in this. For example, patients with Lewy body dementia have considerably greater impairment of attention compared with patients with other types of dementia and often show fluctuations in attentional function.

Given the centrality of inattention to the definition of delirium, much more needs to be learned about the nature of attentional deficits in both dementia and delirium if criteria for the diagnosis of delirium superimposed on dementia are to be developed further.

The diagnostic challenge in an older person presenting with confusion is to disentangle whether they have delirium, dementia or both. Persistent delirium is also possible.

Determining the risk factors for delirium is important for identifying patients who are most susceptible to incident delirium. Predisposing risk factors for incident delirium appear to be dementia, cognitive impairment, functional impairment, previous delirium and fractures on admission.

Patients with pre-existing functional impairment, therefore, need to be well supported in the hospital setting to reduce the risk of developing delirium or becoming more functionally dependent during hospital admission.

It is also crucial to appreciate the effect of social and environmental stressors. One starting point for this analysis is the perhaps obvious perception that, under ordinary everyday conditions, social and environmental factors are not stressors that are strong enough to cause delirium in a person with a healthy brain, even at an advanced age.

Therefore, 'extraordinary' social and environmental stressors are necessary to produce delirium in a healthy elderly person. Extraordinary environmental stress, such as high temperature, may produce delirium in healthy elderly person.

Marked impairments in focusing and sustaining attention (i.e. the ability to maintain attention to stimuli over time) are considered the hallmark feature of delirium.

Complex attentional impairments may also be found in the early stages of Alzheimer's disease (without delirium), but overall the ability to focus and sustain attention is relatively preserved in the earlier stages of Alzheimer's disease.

It has been shown that sustained, divided and selected attention are compromised in the moderate to severe stages of dementia.

The prevalence of major depressive disorder at any given time in community samples of adults aged 65 and older is thought to range from 1 to 5 per cent in most large-scale epidemiological investigations in the United States and internationally.[7]

Late-life depression is also associated with high suicidal ideation and increased healthcare use.

Care partners of people with depression also are at risk for physical and psychiatric illnesses.

Aspects of care might include:

- care packages for people with dementia that include assessment and monitoring for depression and/or anxiety

- a range of tailored interventions, such as reminiscence therapy, multisensory stimulation, animal-assisted therapy and exercise for people with dementia who have depression and/or anxiety.

Treatment should be started by staff with specialist training, who should follow the NICE clinical guideline 'Depression: management of depression in primary and secondary care'[8] after a careful risk–benefit assessment.

Antidepressant drugs with anticholinergic effects should be avoided because they may adversely affect cognition.

The need for adherence, time to onset of action and risk of withdrawal effects should be explained at the start of treatment.

The role of family and care partners in supporting the health and wellbeing of people with dementia

Those carrying out care partners' assessment should seek to identify any psychological distress and the psychosocial impact on the care partner. This should be an ongoing process and should include any period after the person with dementia has entered residential care.

Care plans for care partners of people with dementia should involve a range of tailored interventions. These may consist of multiple components including:

- individual or group psychoeducation

- peer-support groups with other care partners

- support and information by telephone and through the internet

- training courses about dementia, services and welfare benefits

- involvement of other family members in family meetings.

Active steps should be taken to involve, people with dementia in psychoeducation, support and other meetings for care partners in a meaningful way.

Care partners of people with dementia who experience psychological distress and negative psychological impact should be offered appropriate psychological intervention.

Health and social care managers should ensure that care partners of people with dementia have access to a comprehensive range of respite/short-break services.

Care plans should meet the needs of both the care partner (in terms of location, flexibility and timeliness) and the person with dementia, and should include, for example, day care, day- and night-sitting, adult placement and short-term and/or overnight residential care.

Respite/short-break care of any sort should be characterised by meaningful and therapeutic activity tailored to the person with dementia and provided in an environment that meets their needs. Providing this in the person's own home should be considered whenever possible.

The benefits and limitations of medication to manage behavioural and psychological issues, including associated risks

Psychological and behavioural distress generally represent the expression of 'unmet needs', rather than being an inevitable consequence of dementia.

The distress can often be reduced if the unmet need is identified and met.

If antipsychotics are considered to be justified for the management of behavioural and psychological symptoms of dementia (BPSD), they should be initiated by (or in consultation with) a specialist and used only for short periods.

Low-dose, regularly reviewed risperidone is an option for the treatment of psychosis or for agitation or aggression when the risk of not treating outweighs the potential risks associated with antipsychotics in dementia. Patients with Lewy body dementia and Parkinson's disease dementia are particularly sensitive to the extrapyramidal side effects of antipsychotics and the drugs should not be used without specialist psychiatric advice.

Benzodiazepines have no place in the treatment of people with dementia and their use to treat agitation in patients with dementia can be dangerous.

Memantine and cholinesterase inhibitors are considered to be of no value in improving agitation in people with Alzheimer's disease.

Although some symptoms can be appropriately and safely treated with antipsychotics, a fine balance must be achieved between the benefits of these medications, which are often modest, and adverse events, which may have significant consequences.

Reducing the inappropriate or unnecessary use of antipsychotics among people with dementia has been the focus of increasing attention owing to better awareness of the potential problems associated with these medications and their lack of efficacy for symptoms other than severe aggression or delusions.

Several approaches have been used to reduce use of antipsychotics among persons with dementia, including policy or regulatory changes, public reporting and educational outreach. Recently, there has been encouraging evidence of a downward trend in the use of antipsychotics in many long-term care settings, although prescribing rates are still higher than what is likely optimal.

Advice from secondary care should be sought if considering an antipsychotic for an elderly patient. Elderly people with dementia are at risk from specific serious and life-threatening side effects when treated with antipsychotics. The most important adverse effect associated with antipsychotics is sedation.

Antipsychotics should be commenced at the lowest possible dose, titrated carefully and reviewed within the first four weeks and after 6–12 weeks.

Discontinuation should be considered unless there is severe risk or extreme distress.

Risperidone is the only antipsychotic licensed for the treatment of dementia-related behavioural disturbances and then only specifically for short-term (up to six weeks) treatment of persistent aggression in Alzheimer's dementia unresponsive to non-pharmacological approaches and where there is a risk of harm to the patient or others.

Supporting individuals in undertaking psychosocial interventions

There is increasing attention being given to incorporating non-pharmacological psychosocial interventions in dementia care, which can improve quality of life.

There is an urgent need for more good-quality research in the field.

Validation

Validation therapy is an approach used to communicate with disorientated elderly people that involves acknowledging and supporting their feelings in whatever time and place is real to them, even if this may not correspond to their 'here and now' reality. A Cochrane abstract reads:[9] 'Validation therapy has attracted a good deal of criticism from researchers who dispute the evidence for some of the beliefs and values of validation therapy, and the appropriateness of the techniques.'

Validation therapy focuses on dementia from an emotional, rather than factual, perspective. It is based on the principle that even the most confused behaviour has some meaning for the person.

Purported benefits claimed for patients through the use of validation therapy include:

- restoration of self-worth

- promotion of communication and interaction with other people

- reduction of stress and anxiety.

Counselling and psychotherapy

Sessions involve meeting with and sharing problems with a therapist on an individual basis in a confidential setting. There are different types of counselling and psychotherapy to choose from. The therapist aims to understand the client's particular problems so that they can work to overcome or manage these differently.

Reminiscence therapy

Reminiscence therapy (RT) involves the discussion of past activities, events and experiences, with another person or group of people. This is often assisted by aids such as videos, music, pictures, archives and life story books. RT is one of the most popular psychosocial interventions in dementia care, and is highly rated by staff and participants.

Sensory stimulation

Sensory stimulation refers to different techniques used to stimulate the senses to increase alertness and reduce agitation, as well as to enhance quality of life, which is the overall aim of sensory stimulation methods.

Most sensory stimulation interventions considered are single sensory, while few are multisensory interventions. Single stimulation requires stimulation to only one sensory modality, while multisensory stimulation requires stimulation of two or more senses, within a session.

Supporting people with dementia to access local services and referral pathways, including voluntary and community services which would promote their physical and mental health

Professionals will try to give an individual with dementia and closest family members the information they need.

The complexity of ageing and co-morbidity in dementia

Multi-morbidity is a concept that is very familiar to clinicians. In patients who are unwell, clusters of disease states are common, and recognising which morbidities should be prioritised is a key part of good geriatric clinical care. However, modern medicine has been slow to address the implications of multi-morbidity.

A particular strength of the NICE guideline on multi-morbidity[10] is the more clinically relevant approach taken to the recognition of intrusive multi-morbidity as identified by symptom complexes (e.g. frailty and chronic pain) and burdens (e.g. polypharmacy and need for multiagency support).

New and emerging knowledge of psychosocial approaches that can be used to enhance the wellbeing of people with dementia

Aromatherapy is proposed as a complementary intervention to treat a wide range of health problems, including lack of sleep and behavioural symptoms for people with dementia. Aromatherapy is based on the use of plant products or aromatic plant oils to produce essential oils and blends of aromatic compounds. Aromatherapy can be delivered through massage or topical application, inhalation and water immersion.

Massage and touch therapy have been proposed as non-pharmacological interventions to be used in dementia to offset manifestations of cognitive decline and behavioural disturbances, including related psychological problems such as depression and anxiety, and to improve quality of life. Acupressure is a kind of massage and originates from the Jin and Han dynasty (248–8 BC) in China. Acupressure treatment involves the stimulation of certain acupoints by pressing with the fingers or moving limbs or joints slowly.

Notes

1. Sommerlad, A., Ruegger, J., Singh-Manoux, A., Lewis, G. and Livingston, G. (2017) 'Marriage and risk of dementia: systematic review and meta-analysis of observational studies.' *J Neurol Neurosurg Psychiatry.* doi: 10.1136/jnnp-2017-316274

2. See Crowe, M., Andel, R., Pedersen, N.L., Johansson, B. *et al.* (2003) 'Does participation in leisure activities lead to reduced risk of Alzheimer's disease? A prospective study of Swedish twins.' *Journals of Gerontology Series B: Psychological Sciences and Social Sciences 58B*, 249–255; Scarmeas, N., Levy, G., Tang, M.X., Manly, J. *et al.* (2001) 'Influence of leisure activity on the incidence of Alzheimer's disease.' *Neurology 57*, 2236–2242.

3. Alzheimer Society Manitoba, 'Reducing risk of falls for people with dementia.' Accessed on 4 October at www.alzheimer.mb.ca/wp-content/uploads/2013/09/2014-Dementia-Fall-Risk-Checklist-template.pdf

4. AGS (2002) 'The management of persistent pain in older persons.' *J Am Geriatr Soc 50*, S205–S224; AGS (2009) 'Pharmacological management of persistent pain in older persons.' *Pain Med 10*, 1062–1083.

5. Department of Health (2010) 'How to use Essence of Care.' Accessed on 2 September 2017 at www.gov.uk/government/publications/essence-of-care-2010

6. Russ, T.C., Shenkin, S.D., Reynish, E., Ryan, T. *et al.* (2012) 'Dementia in acute hospital inpatients: the role of the geriatrician.' *Age Ageing 41*, 3, 282–284.

7. Hasin, D.S., Goodwin, R.D., Stinson, F.S. and Grant, B.F. (2005) 'Epidemiology of major depressive disorder: Results from the National Epidemiologic Survey on Alcoholism and Related Conditions.' *Arch Gen Psychiatr 62*, 1097–1106.

8. NICE (2004) Clinical guideline [CG23]. Accessed on 2 September 2017 at www.nice.org.uk/guidance/cg23

9. Neal, M. and Barton Wright, P. (2003) 'Validation therapy for dementia.' *Cochrane Database of Systematic Reviews, 3*, CD001394. Accessed on 4 October 2017 at http://onlinelibrary.wiley.com/doi/10.1002/14651858.CD001394/abstract;jsessionid=B5595E4901E822F05E41B61C1B47C283.f04t01

10. NICE (2016) Guideline [NG56]. Accessed on 2 September 2017 at www.nice.org.uk/guidance/ng56

7

Pharmacological interventions in dementia care

Main classes of drugs used to treat dementia

Research in people with dementia focuses on treatments that prevent or delay dementia onset and/or progression and manage dementia-specific symptoms, such as the neuropsychiatric or behavioural symptoms common in people with dementia. Evidence for the efficacy of these medications is conflicting, and the harms of some, such as antipsychotics and benzodiazepines, make them potentially inappropriate in this population.

Antipsychotics in dementia

Reducing the inappropriate or unnecessary use of antipsychotics among persons with dementia has been the focus of increasing attention owing to better awareness of the limited effectiveness and potential problems associated with these medications.

Antidepressants in dementia

Depression is a frequent and important co-morbidity in dementia, and antidepressants are often used to treat depression.

They are also used to treat other behavioural and psychological symptoms (BPSD) of dementia, including agitation, aggression, psychosis and apathy, yet well-designed trials and systematic reviews of the literature have generally found little or equivocal evidence for the effectiveness of antidepressants in the treatment of depression in dementia or BPSD.

Despite this, individuals with dementia may be prescribed antidepressants. Due to their widespread use in the absence of definitive evidence of their effects and side effects in populations with dementia, it is important to establish their efficacy and tolerability in dementia.

Overall, despite being very commonly used, the evidence for antidepressants having a positive role in depression in people with dementia is weak. Additionally, there is no good evidence that antidepressants are effective in improving other outcomes, such as activities of daily living, cognition, clinical severity or care partner stress.

However, antidepressants have some adverse effects, which are common and sometimes serious. In view of these adverse effects and the absence of evidence for positive effects, they should not be used in people without a history of depression in younger ages, unless psychosocial treatments are unsuccessful.[1]

Anxiolytics in dementia

The treatment of anxiety, like that of depression, follows a 'stepped' care approach. You can help people with dementia with mild anxiety by making time to listen and provide reassurance.

Other ways of helping include making adjustments so that their living environment is calmer and safer, and they have an improved structure to everyday life. People with more severe and persistent anxiety can respond well to psychological therapies, although there is evidence that people with dementia have poorer outcomes with CBT for anxiety. There is also some evidence that music therapy with a qualified therapist reduces agitation, which can be a symptom of anxiety.

It is not advisable to prescribe a person with dementia a benzo-diazepine. Benzodiazepines do not actually improve symptoms of anxiety in these patients anyway.

Anticonvulsants in dementia

Antiepileptic drugs are a class of medications that have received considerable attention as possible treatments for agitation and aggression in patients with dementia. Again, it is important to recognise that there is no good evidence that these drugs are superior to placebo in the management of agitation, aggression or anxiety in people with dementia.

Polypharmacy, inappropriate medication and multi-morbidity

BOX 7.1 NATIONAL OCCUPATIONAL STANDARDS ON PRESCRIBING MEDICATION FOR INDIVIDUALS WITH A LONG-TERM CONDITION

National Occupational Standard SFHCMA7 – 'Prescribe medication for individuals with a long term conditions' – is about prescribing medication to reduce the impact of a long-term condition on individuals' health and wellbeing. It covers relating the prescription to the individual's condition and treatment plan and, where appropriate, making arrangements for repeat prescriptions. This standard is relevant to those who may be responsible for prescribing medication.

People with dementia have as many co-morbidities as their peers (cognitively intact people of a comparable age) and take a mean of five or more medications daily.

However, people with dementia are more likely than their peers to use certain medication classes, such as antihypertensives, laxatives, diuretics, antidepressants and antipsychotics.

This medication use may reflect risk factors for dementia and common co-morbidities such as cardio- and reno-vascular disease.

Age-related pharmacokinetic changes occur in all older people, and an altered blood–brain barrier permeability in people with dementia means that they may be more sensitive to neurological and cognitive effects of medications than their peers. These pharmacokinetic changes are additional to drug–disease interactions that occur in dementia.

After dementia onset, medication appropriateness to manage co-morbidities is complicated by a relative absence of evidence. Preventive treatments may require a treatment time to benefit that exceeds life expectancy, or may target treatment goals that are not relevant to the individual or their families.

Polypharmacy and inappropriate medication use among older adults are known to contribute to adverse drug reactions, falls, cognitive impairment, noncompliance, hospitalisation and mortality. Multi-morbidity and polypharmacy are increasingly prevalent among older people in populations.

While de-prescribing – the act of tapering, reducing or stopping a medication – has been shown in small studies to be feasible and relatively safe, clinicians continue to find it difficult to stop medications. Barriers include difficulty making decisions to stop medications (both from the clinician and patient perspective), worry about stopping medications started by others, limited knowledge about how to stop medications, and concern about medication withdrawal effects.

The importance of recording and reporting side effects and/or adverse reactions to medication

If a patient thinks he or she may have had a side effect as a reaction to one of your medicines, he or she can report this online on the Yellow Card Scheme.[2] The Yellow Card Scheme is used to make pharmacists, doctors and nurses aware of any new side effects that medicines or any other healthcare products may have caused.

If you wish to report a side effect, you will need to provide basic information about:

- the side effect
- the name of the medicine that you think caused it
- the person who had the side effect
- your contact details as the reporter of the side effect.

It is helpful if you have to hand the medication and/or the leaflet that came with it while you fill out the report.

The importance of recording/reporting side effects/adverse reactions can be summarised thus:

- increased awareness of the individual's condition
- accurate judgements can be made
- able to use the individual's history to make judgements
- monitoring clinical changes
- monitoring the safety of medicines.

Cognitive enhancers

It is likely that the development of cognitive enhancers in the future for Alzheimer's disease will vary according to when they are most effective in the time-course of the disease and when a diagnosis can be reliably made. This might even be before the 'official' onset of symptoms.

There is an ethical debate still to be had fully about this.

Figure 7.1 shows four possible points in time for intervention.

Sadly, currently, the diagnosis is often not made at all, or made very late in the process, by which time cognitive impairment, disability and behavioural symptoms may be all quite marked (T4 in Figure 7.1). One aim may therefore be to advance the time at which the diagnosis is made to the earliest stage possible using current routinely available diagnostic technologies and health system structures (T2). Researchers have qualified this aim by proposing that we should aim for 'timely' rather than 'early' diagnosis, responding to concerns raised by older people and family members (T3) rather than 'screening' older populations proactively for early signs and symptoms.

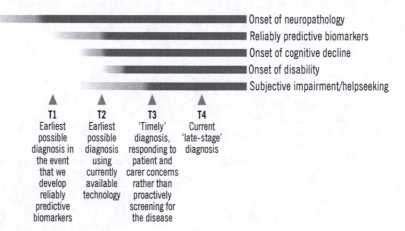

Figure 7.1 Timeline
Source: Reproduced by kind permission of Alzheimer's Disease International, from 'World Alzheimer Report 2011: The benefits of early diagnosis and intervention', p.11.[3]

Cholinergic hypothesis of Alzheimer's disease

An initial breakthrough in Alzheimer's disease came in the 1970s with the demonstration of a cholinergic deficit in the brains of patients with Alzheimer's disease, mediated by deficits of the enzyme choline acetyltransferase.

The cholinergic hypothesis was the first theory proposed to explain Alzheimer's disease and has since led to the development of the main class of drugs currently approved to treat mild to moderate Alzheimer's disease.

This theory was based on the finding that a loss of cholinergic activity is commonly observed in the *post-mortem* brains of patients with

Alzheimer's disease, and experimental studies in humans and non-human primates have suggested a role for acetylcholine (ACh) in learning and memory. These studies reported that by blocking central cholinergic activity with scopolamine, young subjects would demonstrate memory deficits similar to those seen in aged individuals.

This theory led to early acetylcholinesterase inhibitors clinical studies utilising another type of cholinergic agonist, acetylcholinesterase inhibitors (AChEIs) that initially showed promise in reversing the memory impairment in patients with Alzheimer's disease.

This, along with the recognition of the role of acetylcholine in memory and learning, led to the cholinergic hypothesis of Alzheimer's disease and stimulated attempts to therapeutically increase cholinergic activity.

Cholinergic depletion is thought to be a feature of the neuro-degenerative cascade. Cholinesterase inhibitors block the cholinesterase enzyme, which breaks down acetyl choline at the synaptic cleft, potentiating cholinergic transmission.

Taken together, these studies show that AChEIs can provide small amounts of symptomatic improvement but offer no long-term cure for this disorder. The average benefit experienced by a patient with Alzheimer's disease who is started on one of these drugs is only modest and is approximately of the order of one MMSE point in magnitude. However, the effect is sustained, even as patients become more severely affected by dementia. Although the drugs don't slow down progression, the modest improvements of cognitive and functional abilities are measurable and are considered to represent a significant benefit for some and to represent a meaningful difference in wellbeing.

Drug therapy

Pharmacological treatment consists of cognitive enhancers, including the cholinesterase inhibitors (donepezil, galantamine and rivastigmine), and memantine, an N-methyl-D-aspartic acid receptor antagonist. The basic evidence to support the use of these drugs remains unchanged and, in general, the costs of the drugs are now significantly lower, particularly for donepezil.

One of the following is usually recommended: donepezil, galantamine and rivastigmine for people with mild or moderate dementia of the Alzheimer type, providing that:

- the medicine is started by a specialist in the care of people with dementia

- a person receiving treatment has regular reviews and assessments of their condition. (Reviews are usually carried out by a specialist team. Care partners' views on the person's condition should also be sought before the medicine is started and should be considered during the reviews.)

There is little to choose between acetylcholinesterase inhibitors (AChEIs). Price and tolerability are the key deciders. The main side effects of AChEIs are syncope and gastrointestinal upset and they are contraindicated in heart block, significant cardiac conduction problems or if the pulse rate is <60.

Memantine is an alternative, if cardiac problems preclude an AChEI, and also has a licence for use in severe dementia, but it is more expensive. Renal function needs to be checked before prescribing. Consideration of memantine should generally involve a specialist.

Memantine can be considered as a treatment option for:

- people who have moderate Alzheimer's disease and who, for some reason, cannot take, or are intolerant to, the acetylcholinesterase inhibitor medicines

- people who have severe Alzheimer's disease (but it is not as good as a cholinesterase inhibitor in severe Alzheimer's disease).

Most people with mild to moderate Alzheimer's disease will respond to and derive valuable benefits from one of the AChEIs or, as an alternative in moderate to severe disease, memantine. Their use is recommended by NICE.[4]

Systematic follow-up is needed, but not necessarily in a specialist hospital clinic. AChEIs should be continued, even when dementia enters the more severe stages, providing they are well tolerated.

Much of the research effort in the dementia of the Alzheimer type in the last decade has been directed towards disease-modifying therapy that could alter the course of the disease rather than act on symptoms alone. However, the lack of effective disease-modifying drugs arising from these studies reflects the challenges involved in developing a therapeutic agent with the potential to modify the course of a disease as complex as Alzheimer's disease. There is general agreement that anticholinergic burden should be minimised in those with dementia, especially before prescribing cholinergic medication.

Anticholinergic use has been associated with poorer cognitive and functional performance, cognitive decline and with increased risk for dementia. Scales to assess anticholinergic burden are available.

However, higher cholinesterase inhibitor (ChEI) doses, regardless of drug agent, can be associated with better longitudinal cognitive and functional capacities. Although the target organ for these drugs is the brain, the heart is also rich in cholinesterases and their inhibition may adversely affect cardiac function. These cardiac adverse effects, including bradycardia, heart block and QT prolongation with or without a history of cardiac disease, can emerge as vagotonic effects due to ChEIs. (You should always consult an authoritative source of knowledge, such as the *British National Formulary*.)

Approved drug treatments
Cholinesterase inhibitors
Tacrine was the first-generation cholinesterase inhibitor but was limited by hepatotoxic side effects. Donepezil, rivastigmine and galantamine then followed, with the former probably the most widely used agent.

Efficacy appears similar between these different agents, so choice should be based on cost, individual patient tolerance and physician experience.

Donepezil is prescribed at an initial dose of 5 mg in the evening, increased to 10 mg after one month if appropriate.

The UK Donepezil and Memantine in Moderate to Severe AD (DOMINO) study,[5] which randomised those on stable donepezil with moderate to severe dementia to continuation donepezil, discontinuation, a change to memantine or adding memantine, clearly showed that continued donepezil treatment (or a switch to memantine or combination therapy) was associated with cognitive and functional benefits over the following 12 months, compared with placebo.

The three acetylcholinesterase inhibitors donepezil, galantamine and rivastigmine are recommended as options in the management of people with Alzheimer's disease of moderate severity only (i.e. those with a MMSE score of between 10 and 20 points), and under the following conditions.

Only specialists in the care of people with dementia (i.e. psychiatrists including those specialising in learning disability, neurologists and physicians specialising in the care of the elderly) should initiate treatment. Care partners' views on the patient's condition at baseline should be sought.

Common side effects are gastrointestinal, fatigue and muscle cramps. Care should be taken if considering commencing a cholinesterase inhibitor in a person with a history of peptic or duodenal ulcer disease. Small numbers of patients may exhibit an acute worsening of cognition or agitation on starting.

Post-hoc analyses of randomised controlled trial data might in future indicate some benefit in specific populations characterised by the presence of biomarkers.[6]

Memantine

Memantine uncompetitively blocks the NMDA receptor and, thus, may theoretically be neuroprotective by preventing neuron loss, as well as improving symptoms by helping to restore function of damaged neurons.

Memantine is initially prescribed at a dose of 5 mg daily, increasing weekly by 5 mg to a maximum dose of 20 mg. It is generally well tolerated, with fewer side effects than cholinesterase inhibitors, although dizziness, headache, somnolence, constipation and hypertension can occur.

Memantine has been shown to have modest benefits in moderate to severe Alzheimer's disease, with little evidence supporting its use in milder Alzheimer's disease.

Additionally, the addition of memantine to donepezil monotherapy may be beneficial in those with mid-stage Alzheimer's disease. Neither memantine nor donepezil are beneficial in mild cognitive impairment.

While these medications represent our best current available pharmacological treatments in Alzheimer's disease, they have relatively small average overall effect and do not alter the course of the underlying neurodegenerative process.

It is likely that the down regulation of cholinergic transmission occurs too far downstream in this process for treatments such as cholinesterase inhibitors to exhibit such an effect.

With this in mind, targeting the pathological process 'upstream' has also been the focus of much attention.

Drugs for dementia with Lewy bodies

Pharmacological management of dementia with Lewy bodies (DLB) remains one of the most challenging issues facing all clinicians.

The combination of cognitive, neuropsychiatric, autonomic and motor features in DLB is, when compared with Alzheimer's disease, much more likely to lead to greater functional impairment and poorer quality of life.

Early randomised controlled trials of the ChEI rivastigmine demonstrated benefit in cognition in diffuse Lewy body dementia and Parkinson's disease dementia, and also showed effects upon neuropsychiatric symptoms.

Vascular dementia

There has been a suggestion that cholinergic dysfunction occurs in vascular dementia, prompting interest in the use of ChEIs for this disorder.

In clinical practice, many patients given a diagnosis of vascular dementia or mixed vascular and Alzheimer's dementia will actually have significant amounts of Alzheimer pathology in their brains and may show a reasonable response to a cholinesterase inhibitor.

Where prevention of recurrent stroke is necessary, use of anti-hypertensive therapy in the case of haemorrhagic stroke and use of antiplatelets or anticoagulants, antihypertensive and lipid-lowering strategies after ischaemic stroke according to national guidelines should be implemented.

The range of drugs to manage behavioural and psychological symptoms of dementia and when such drugs should or should not be used

Behavioural and psychological symptoms of dementia (BPSD) are manifestations of need and may be markers of distress. The first approach is to understand the need and try to address it. So, for example, underlying pain and infection must be sought and treated, and care partners should be trained and supported.

In 2009, the UK Department of Health commissioned a policy review on antipsychotic use in dementia. The resulting report concluded that usage was unacceptably high and recommended a two-thirds reduction over a period of three years as a target.[7]

Current advice is as follows:

> If a person with Lewy body dementia (dementia with Lewy bodies or Parkinson's disease dementia) is prescribed an antipsychotic drug, it should be done with the utmost care, under constant supervision and with regular review. This is because people with Lewy body dementia, who often have visual hallucinations, are at particular risk of severe adverse (negative) reactions to antipsychotics.[8]

There is a relatively small range of drugs that can be used and drugs should not be the first option.

If antipsychotics are considered to be justified for the management of BPSD, they should be initiated by (or in consultation with) a specialist and used only for short periods.

Only one antipsychotic drug, risperidone, is licensed for treatment of dementia-related behavioural disturbances in the UK, and then only specifically for short-term treatment (up to six weeks) of persistent aggression in moderate to severe Alzheimer's dementia unresponsive to non-pharmacological approaches and where there is risk of harm to the patient or others.

The risperidone licence for the short-term treatment of persistent aggression in Alzheimer's dementia was granted in 2008 after a new analysis of three randomised controlled trials conducted on behavioural problems in the elderly showed a clear benefit for the short- term use of risperidone when aggression only was considered.[9]

Antipsychotics can be potentially fatal in Alzheimer's disease, Lewy body dementia and Parkinson's disease dementia and should not be used without specialist psychiatric advice.

Antipsychotic medications are often used to treat behavioural and psychological symptoms of dementia. Antipsychotics have been widely prescribed for BPSD since the 1960s, partly inferring potential efficacy for the treatment of psychotic symptoms not only because of the benefit in treating psychosis in the context of schizophrenia and bipolar disorder, but also because of their sedative properties. The use of typical antipsychotics has declined to some degree, but they are still widely used.

Although the use of typical antipsychotics has declined, atypical antipsychotic drugs remain, however, the first-line pharmacological treatment for BPSD in most countries.

Available evidence indicates that risperidone, olanzapine and aripiprazole exhibit modest benefits in the management of aggression and psychosis over a 6–12-week period in individuals with Alzheimer's disease.[10] In addition, there is limited evidence for the use of these medications in individuals with non-AD-type dementia. Furthermore, the benefit of using antipsychotics as a longer-term treatment in individuals with dementia is unclear.

The use of antipsychotics in the management of psychotic symptoms and aggression in individuals with dementia must be balanced against their serious adverse effects profile. Antipsychotic use increases the risk for death, cerebrovascular adverse events, Parkinsonism, sedation, gait disturbance, cognitive decline and pneumonia. Given the significant risk for mortality when antipsychotics are used in individuals with dementia, the US Food and Drug Administration (FDA), the European Medicines Agency and the UK Medicines and Healthcare Products Regulatory Agency have all issued warnings regarding their use in individuals with dementia.

Numerous reviews have evaluated the use of antipsychotics in individuals with dementia. However, none of these reviews have systematically studied the data on the use of antipsychotics in individuals with dementia exclusively from meta-analyses. Systematic reviews and meta-analyses of well-designed and completed randomised controlled trials can provide the highest levels of evidence to support therapeutic interventions.

Ethical issues around drug treatments in the care of people living with dementia

Inappropriate over-prescribing of antipsychotic medication is recognised as a marker of poor care, especially if prescriptions are not regularly reviewed by the prescribing physician.

Although the principle of protecting older people's human rights when they cannot consent to treatment is well developed with respect to the use of physical restraints and deprivation of liberty, it is acknowledged that protection against inappropriate use of 'chemical restraints' is relatively less well developed.

To date, controlled trials have demonstrated limited clinical efficacy for use of antipsychotics in BPSD, with only small effect sizes reported on global behavioural disturbance and specific behavioural symptoms.

Long-term use of antipsychotic drugs is also associated with increasing concerns about serious adverse effects including mortality.

New and emerging knowledge of pharmacological interventions that can be used to enhance the wellbeing of people with dementia

Studies of potentially disease-modifying therapy up to now have generally been undertaken in patients with clinically detectable, established disease, while mounting evidence suggests that the pathological changes associated with dementia begin to occur several years before the emergence of the clinical syndrome.

It is possible, then, that pharmacological therapy may be more beneficial in this pre-clinical stage before the neurodegenerative process has been established.

Techniques to provide earlier diagnosis are key to testing this theory in clinical trials, facilitating trials in pre-symptomatic phases.

BOX 7.2 NOVEL THERAPIES

Anti-amyloid therapy

These agents generally have three different target sites: directly targeting Aβ, and either the gamma or beta-secretase enzymes involved in APP cleavage.

Beta-secretase enzyme

Small molecule beta-secretase inhibitors have demonstrated reduced CSF beta-amyloid compared to controls.

Gamma-secretase enzyme

e.g. Trials of semagacestat and tarenflurbil

Immunisation

e.g. Active immunisation against Aβ

Tau-targeted therapy

Tau-targeted strategies that are, at the time of writing, in clinical trials include agents to prevent hyperphosphorylation, as well as those targeting microtubule stability and aggregation.

Notes

1. An extremely important contribution was the 'Lancet Commission' on dementia: Livingston, G., Sommerlad, A., Orgeta, V., Costafreda, S.G. *et al.* (2017) 'Dementia prevention, intervention, and care.' *Lancet S0140-6736*, 17, 31363–31366. doi: http://dx.doi.org/10.1016/S0140-6736(17)31363-6

2. See the Yellow Card website, accessed on 2 September 2017 at www.mhra.gov.uk/yellowcard

3. Accessed on 4 October 2017 at www.alz.co.uk/research/WorldAlzheimerReport2011.pdf

4. NICE (2011) 'Donezipil, galantamine, rivastigmine and memantine for the treatment of Alzheimer's disease.' Technology appraisal guidance [TA217]. Accessed on 4 October 2017 at www.nice.org.uk/guidance/ta217/chapter/1-guidance

5. Howard, R., McShane, R., Lindesay, J., Ritchie, C. *et al.* (2012) 'Donepezil and memantine for moderate-to-severe Alzheimer's disease.' *New England Journal of Medicine 366*, 10, 893–903, doi: 10.1056/NEJMoa1106668

6. For example, Murray, M.E., Kouri, N., Lin, W.L., Jack, C.R. Jr, Dickson, D.W. and Vemuri, P. (2014) 'Clinicopathologic assessment and imaging of tauopathies in neurodegenerative dementias.' *Alzheimer's Research and Therapy 6*, 1, 1.

7. Banerjee, S. (2009) 'The use of antipsychotic medicine for people with dementia: Time for action.' An independent report commissioned and funded by the Department of Health. Accessed on 4 October 2017 at www.rcpsych.ac.uk/pdf/Antipsychotic%20Bannerjee%20Report.pdf

8. https://www.alzheimers.org.uk/info/20162/drugs/106/drugs_used_to_relieve_behavioral_and_psychological_symptoms/5

9. European Medicines Agency approval. Accessed on 8 November 2017 at www.ema.europa.eu/ema/index.jsp?curl=pages/medicines/human/referrals/Risperdal/human_referral_000022.jsp

10. See, for example, Liperoti, R., Pedone, C. and Corsonello, A. (2008) 'Antipsychotics for the treatment of behavioural and psychological symptoms of dementia (BPSD).' *Current Neuropharmacology 6*, 2, 117–124. Accessed on 4 October 2017 at www.ncbi.nlm.nih.gov/pmc/articles/PMC2647149

8

Living well with dementia and promoting independence

The importance of physical activity (including access to outside space) in maintaining a person's independence and abilities

Care partners have identified physical function as an important component of quality of life for their care recipients with dementia.

The importance of maintaining mobility and physical activity in dementia has been recognised in clinical and long-term care settings, and randomised trials have demonstrated that individualised exercise programmes are both feasible and beneficial for increasing strength and maintaining mobility for cognitively impaired nursing home residents.[1]

However, to date, randomised clinical trials of community-based interventions to promote physical activity in older adults have typically excluded individuals with cognitive impairment, either through explicit criteria or because such individuals are unable to successfully complete the programmes and/or assessments.

Supporting individuals to meet their daily living needs

Coping with dementia is considered extremely difficult because of the often unpredictable and difficult-to-understand changes that accompany the disease. The progressive nature of dementia makes it even more challenging to adjust to emergent changes, and makes coping with and adjusting to the disease a cyclic and continuing process.

Although people with dementia try to maintain a normal life as long as possible, they also have to deal with the expected deterioration and the fear of losing their intellectual and social competencies.

Supporting individuals to continue their interests, social life and community involvement, and why this is important

Domestic-type activities could be encouraged and reminiscence used to promote feelings of worth – for example, setting tables, watering gardens.

A range of activities should be provided that can adapt as the dementia progresses or other health-related factors intervene – for example, music therapy, cooking, art and sensory experiences.

Community involvement should be encouraged – for example, concerts, outings, schoolchildren visits, service club involvement, day centre visits.

People living with dementia should be encouraged and given the opportunity to continue their social roles where possible.

Tactile stimulation through craft, touching or feeling items, tasting food items or smelling flowers may be useful in reminiscing and provide pleasure. All activity should allow for maximum independence and be paced according to the person's capabilities.

The person's preferred language should be established and clearly documented. Daily conversations in the person's preferred language should be conducted by using an interpreter or a worker or care partner who speaks the same language, or by using visitor schemes, church groups, clubs or friends.

Books, including picture books, in the person's preferred language should be available.

Community initiatives such as the development of dementia-friendly environments

Neighbourhood plays an active role in the lives of people with dementia, setting limits and constraints but also offering significant opportunities, encompassing forms of help and support as yet rarely discussed in the field of dementia studies.

To ensure a better life for this rising number of individuals with dementia and their families, consumers, policy makers and researchers around the world have begun exploring and embracing the concept of 'dementia-friendly communities'.

A policy initiative, which was one of the three areas of action outlined in the 'Prime Minister's Challenge on Dementia', encourages cities, towns and villages to sign up to become more dementia-friendly.[2]

The Alzheimer's Society programmes on 'dementia-friendly communities' was established under the aforementioned policy initiative to facilitate the creation and recognition of dementia-friendly communities across the country. The recognition process of the Alzheimer Society enables communities to be publicly recognised for their work towards becoming dementia-friendly.[3]

> A dementia-friendly community should be a place where there is increased awareness that dementia is a disease that touches the lives of many, and so requires community-based solutions. Greater awareness will, in turn, support better diagnosis rates and joined-up working by health and social care providers.[4]

The starting point was the Alzheimer's Society 'DFCsurvey', to which over 500 people with dementia responded, and the invaluable evidence provided in interviews with people with dementia and their care partners.

Although there are some excellent examples of communities gearing up for dementia, many people with dementia do not feel supported and a part of their local area.

- Less than half of the respondents to the DFCsurvey thought that their area is geared up to help them live well with dementia (42%).

- Less than half feel a part of the community (47%). Results become considerably lower the more advanced the person's dementia is.

- Nearly three-quarters (73%) of UK adults surveyed in the YouGov poll do not think that society is geared up to deal with dementia.[4]

Even within the context of 'communities working towards becoming dementia-friendly', the definitions of 'dementia-friendly' and 'community' remain diverse. The concept of 'dementia-friendly' may refer to individuals with dementia (IWD), or refer to both IWD and their care partners. Even though most would agree that a critical way to support IWD is to support their care partners, many insist that IWD should remain central when defining 'dementia-friendly'.

To add to another level of complexity, the concept of 'community' may represent a place, the social and physical environments, an organisation, a group of individuals, a society, a culture or virtual communities.

What 'community' means to one person may be completely different from another.

Additionally, as the interpretation of 'dementia-friendly' can be shaped by the political, social, cultural, historical, economic, moral and other factors that surround a community, so are the defining attributes of 'dementia-friendly'.

For example, in one definition, the defining attributes of 'dementia-friendly' are empowerment, aspiration, self-confidence, contribution, participation and meaningful activities.[5] These attributes may imply that the purposes of becoming dementia-friendly are to acknowledge the 'personhood' of IWD, and to sustain their sense of meaning in life.

In another definition, the essential attributes of 'dementia-friendly' include wayfinding ability, a sense of safety, accessibility to local facilities, social acceptance and understanding of dementia.[6] The emphasis on community accessibility and social acceptance may represent the view of dementia as a type of disability.

Lastly, the attributes of 'dementia-friendly' in a final definition are similar to both others, but with an additional attention to human rights.[7] This attention to human rights may reflect an influence from the Scottish government's view on dementia, that IWD and their care partners have the rights to participation, accountability, non-discrimination and equity, empowerment and legality.

Dementia-friendly environments

The objective of empowering people with dementia by recognising their rights and capabilities so that they feel respected and, to the extent that they are able, empowered to take decisions about their lives is pivotal. This approach believes that the challenge is to create a society where dementia is normalised and people with dementia are supported to continue to live fulfilling lives for as long as possible with the understanding that dementia is a disability.

BOX 8.1 NATIONAL OCCUPATIONAL STANDARDS ON ENVIRONMENTS

National Occupational Standard MH66.2013 – 'Assess how environments and practices can be maintained and improved to promote mental health' – involves identifying all those with a stake in the environments and practices, and consulting with them about their requirements and expectations. These environments may be, for example: homes, workplaces, public places, the broader environment such as towns, housing estates and the countryside, or even social, cultural and aesthetic aspects as well as physical aspects and the interaction of people with their environment. The term 'practices' is used to describe significant activities which take place within the environment.

In institutional settings, residents often experience the environment as restrictive and confining. The environment needs to be able to support remaining ability rather than operate to diminish it, and to support the development and maintenance of relationships. Thus, design of buildings, if regarded as a therapeutic resource, can promote wellbeing and functioning of people with dementia.

It is argued that a 'dementia-friendly environment' should compensate for disability and consider both the importance for the person with dementia of his/her experiences within the environment and also the social, physical and organisational environments which have an impact on these experiences.

The needs of individuals for day-to-day closeness with others (e.g. sharing thoughts and feelings)

A shift in focus from symptoms and disability towards the capacity and potential of the person with dementia is urgently needed to create a more balanced view of dementia and a more dementia-friendly society, which enables people and their families to adapt to the changes dementia brings in their lives and to live well with the condition.

The relatively new concept of social health seems helpful to make such a shift. Social health acknowledges that the person can experience wellbeing despite a medical condition by maintaining a dynamic balance between opportunities and limitations in the context of social and environmental challenges.

Experiencing social health is important not only for the person with dementia but also for their family who often provide care at home and have to deal with major challenges.

One of the crucial elements of implementing shared decision-making in nursing homes appeared to be good communication and relationships between staff and families, as well as a positive attitude of family members.

An excellent example of an intervention that promotes social health is the Meeting Centres Support Programme.[8] A key element of the programme is that it gives support to people with dementia and their care partners in local community centres to promote social participation and integration in the community. This can provide insights into which approaches are the most useful for people with dementia to increase their social participation.

People with dementia describe social relationships as valuable and emphasise the need for social support to be able to cope with their disease. Furthermore, maintaining a sense of mutuality is reported to be essential for spouses to be able to continue caregiving during the dementia process.

Continued closeness in the relationship appears to be crucial to prevent spousal care partners from feeling frustrated. Caring is often described as more fulfilling when spousal care partners maintain their closeness to their partner. To maintain their connection, couples highlight commitment, mutual support and doing things together as essential.

How to recognise and respond to the cultural, spiritual and sexual needs of people with dementia

'This is me' is a simple form for anyone receiving professional care who is living with dementia or is experiencing delirium or other communication difficulties. It is suitable for use in any setting – at home, in hospital, in respite care or a care home and provides a valuable way of integrating person-centred care.[9]

It provides an easy and practical way of recording who the person is. The form includes space to include details on the person's cultural and family background; events, people and places from their lives; preferences and routines; and their personality.

Spiritual care is not, as such, confined to religious beliefs and observance, although religion may be an important part of the person's spiritual needs. There are many different ways to express spirituality – for example, meditating, listening to music, praying, walking in the garden, visiting a favourite place – and people living with dementia should be encouraged to express themselves in their own individual way if possible.

BOX 8.2 NATIONAL OCCUPATIONAL STANDARDS
ON SUPPORTING SPIRITUAL WELLBEING

National Occupational Standard SCDHSC0350 – 'Support the spiritual well-being of individuals' – outlines the requirements to promote, recognise, respect and support individuals' spiritual wellbeing. This includes identifying ways to support individuals' spiritual wellbeing and providing opportunities that facilitate and support this. It also includes evaluating and reporting on work that relates to spiritual wellbeing.

A loving relationship between two people can continue if both are happy to do so. Disinhibited sexual behaviour should be discouraged with sensitivity. This may indicate an unmet need for sexual expression and ways of meeting this need appropriately should be explored.

In a residential setting, sexual expression may be facilitated by the provision of privacy, appropriate furnishings (e.g. double bed) and permitting overnight stays.

The role of family and care partners in enabling people with dementia to live well

In general, informal care partners encounter a variety of problems in a range of different areas; however, a greater number and more complex problems are experienced when the person they are caring for is cognitively impaired (such as in dementia).

Informal care partners describe their task of taking care of a person with dementia as stressful and difficult, especially when behavioural problems are present.

Dementia not only affects people with dementia and their informal care partners directly, but also has an impact on the relationship between a person with dementia and his or her informal care partner.

Particularly, spouses report various changes in the relationship with their partner with dementia. Negative changes are reported in areas such as reciprocity, communication, opportunities for shared activities, and happiness in the relationship.

However, some positive aspects of the relationship are often reported to remain intact, such as closeness and affection.

How activities can be adapted to suit an individual's changing needs

Core to the public health agenda for people with dementia and their care partners is the promotion of wellbeing. Wellbeing concerns the positive aspects of an individual's mental health such as enjoyment and fulfilling one's potential.

To help promote wellbeing among people with dementia, they can be facilitated to participate in meaningful activities in both informal and formal settings. Informally, this may take the form of memory cafes and groups organised for peer support, reading or 'singing for the brain'.

Formally, psychological therapies may be available such as reminiscence therapy, where people with dementia are prompted to recall past events and personal memories.

Because many people with dementia lack the cognitive skills necessary to seek out successfully meaningful activities independently, it is especially important that care partners and residential facilities provide them with such opportunities.

BOX 8.3 NATIONAL OCCUPATIONAL STANDARDS ON THERAPEUTIC GROUP ACTIVITIES

National Occupational Standard SCDHSC0393 – 'Promote participation in agreed therapeutic group activities' – identifies the requirements when you promote participation in agreed therapeutic group activities. This includes planning and preparing activities, preparing and supporting individuals to participate in the activities and contributing to the evaluation of the activities.

Strategies to reduce the struggle with unfamiliar environments

People living with dementia are found in high numbers in the community, in assisted living and in residential settings. Interventions to help individuals find their way in complex environments are important for their safety and autonomy.

Environments such as senior residential buildings (independent-living residences, assisted-living residences and skilled-nursing facilities)

are particularly challenging for wayfinding due to the design of long corridors often with equally spaced doors, a lack of distinctiveness of different areas of the buildings, poor visibility into the distance and poor environmental cues.

Wayfinding systems are designed around what we know about spatial cognition and navigation in humans and other animals. In particular, it has long been recognised that a part of the brain called the hippocampus may be especially important. This part of the brain also tends to be affected quite early on in the neuropathological process of Alzheimer's disease.

Care homes should make use of appropriate signage as this helps people to find their way around.

Meaningful symbols and signifiers used around the home can help people to locate particular rooms and objects more easily. For example, a sponge or facecloth on the bathroom door acts as a prompt as to the room's purpose.

In care homes and group accommodation with many similar doors, numbering or pictures can help some people to identify their own rooms more easily.

Salient cues can enhance memory by providing environmental support for encoding and retrieval so that there is less demand on processing resources.

However, there is relatively little known about the properties of cues or landmarks that make them helpful for wayfinding in older adults with and without dementia who live in residential facilities.

BOX 8.4 NATIONAL OCCUPATIONAL STANDARDS ON COLLABORATING IN THE ASSESSMENT OF NEED FOR SOCIAL SUPPORT

National Occupational Standard SFHGEN75 – SQA Code HC9T 04 – 'Collaborate in the assessment of the need for, and the provision of, environmental and social support in the community' – is concerned with the provision of equipment and support to individuals and care partners in the community.

Ways to adapt the physical environment to promote independence, privacy, orientation and safety (e.g. to reduce risk of falls)

Safety, security, monitoring and reassurance tools can technologically support the safety and monitoring of people with dementia.

They include options to set off alarms in the case of emergency (alarm and pager units, fall detectors, flood detectors, water temperature monitors, lighting) and thereby aim to support the wellbeing, independence and security of the person with dementia as well as to provide reassurance to care partners.

Some areas that could be included in promoting an environment free of falls are shown in Box 8.5.

BOX 8.5 DEMENTIA-FRIENDLY HOUSING

Flooring – non-slip surfaces; prompt cleaning of spills and urine; quick-dry and low-shine cleaning methods; avoidance of flooring patterns that create the illusion of slopes or steps for people with visual impairment; visible highlighting of steps.

Lighting – adequate and even lighting, including stairs; avoidance of glare; wayfinding night lighting to the toilet; making sure night lighting is used consistently and safely.

Threats to mobilising – promptly reducing clutter and other trip hazards in patients' rooms and wards; installing handrails; prompt assessment for walking aids of the correct height and type and that are well maintained and kept within easy reach.

Footwear – unsafe footwear can further compound fall risk, especially in those with gait, balance, lower-limb and proprioceptive problems.

In addition, a failure to act on environmental hazards is not only a risk in itself, but is likely to demotivate staff and adversely affect any other efforts for fall prevention.

Perceptual distortions that may occur in dementia and how the impact of such distortion can be minimised by changes to the environment

Traditional hospital ward environments were not designed to promote independence or to support patients with perceptual and visuospatial difficulties, and yet these are prominent symptoms in the most common types of dementia.

Therefore, negotiating environments with poor lighting, signage, clutter and white walls, ceilings and floors may be difficult for patients with dementia.

For example, patients with dementia can find it difficult to navigate around a hospital ward due to the repetitive décor.

The impact of this 'negative environment' for patients with dementia is the likelihood of increased agitation, confusion and distress, and a reduction in mobility and social interactions, leading to a risk of further health complications.

The principles, processes and options for self-directed support

Direct payments for care were officially introduced in 1996.

There is clear and persistent evidence from research over 20 years of existence that, when used to employ their own personal assistants (rather than use regulated services), and their payments are large enough to meet leisure and social needs as well as personal care needs, people enjoy much better outcomes.

BOX 8.6 NATIONAL OCCUPATIONAL STANDARDS ON SUPPORTING PEOPLE OVER FINANCIAL AFFAIRS

National Occupational Standard SCDHSC0345 – 'Support individuals to manage their financial affairs' – identifies the requirements when supporting individuals to manage their financial affairs. This includes working with individuals to access information and advice, and supporting them to manage their financial affairs.

National Occupational Standard SCDHSC0346 – 'Support individuals to manage direct payments' – outlines the requirements when supporting individuals to access and use direct payments. This includes enabling individuals to access information on direct payments and manage their use.

Self-directed support is available to most people (including people with dementia) who have been assessed by a social worker or other professional as needing help from social work and/or housing.

It allows service users to plan and organise their own care in ways that suit them – bearing in mind other help from family members, friends and neighbours.

Instead of the social work department arranging service users' services and paying for them, the department can give service users directly the money that would have been spent on these services. Recipients can then use this money to pay for the support needed, at the right time and place. This option is called a direct payment.

Service users can use this direct payment to:

- buy support from any service provider such as a private care agency or a voluntary organisation

- employ someone as a personal assistant

- buy services from a local authority if they sell their services.

Service users can also use the direct payment to buy equipment to help with mobility or other needs.

The Wanless Review of social care funding, published in March 2006, noted that the majority of direct payments spend was on personal assistants.[10]

However, practitioners have for some time reported that most service users do not wish to have the responsibility of managing staff and their own support.

Dementia-specific advice and guidance on adapting the physical and social environment to ensure physical safety and emotional security

BOX 8.7 NATIONAL OCCUPATIONAL STANDARDS ON CO-PRODUCTION

National Occupational Standard MH68.2013 – 'Co-produce action plans which assist stakeholders in improving environments and practices to promote mental health' – covers gaining the support of people who use services and other stakeholders and working co-productively to improve environments and practices and facilitating action to do so.

The term 'co-production' refers to a way of working whereby citizens and decision makers, or people who use services, significant others, family care partners and service providers work together to create a decision or service which works for them all. Co-production should entail equal and reciprocal relationships, and not constitute a tokenistic 'box-ticking involvement exercise'.

The approach is value-driven and built on the principle that those who use a service are best placed to help design it.

The introduction of assistive technology to support self-care and meaningful activity

In UK healthcare there are many claims of the benefits of person-centred approaches to health and care.

The majority of older adults want to continue living independently and technologies may enable them to stay in their own home longer before moving to nursing facilities.

Engaging people in their own healthcare is described as a way to improve people's knowledge; enhance people's experience of services; change service use and cost; and positively impact on people's health.

'Assistive technologies' is a catch-all term for any 'device or system that allows an individual to perform a task that they would otherwise be unable to do, or increases the ease and safety with which the task can be performed'.[11]

A subtype of assistive technology is telecare, which usually involves the remote monitoring of people living in their own homes, communicating with them at a distance via telephony and the internet. These are devices used to facilitate independence and enhance personal safety. Telecare includes community alarms, sensors and movement detectors, and the use of video conferencing to communicate with care partners.

BOX 8.8 NATIONAL OCCUPATIONAL STANDARDS ON ASSISTIVE DEVICES/TECHNOLOGIES

National Occupational Standard SFHCHS239 – SQA Code HDOA 04 – 'Enable individuals to use assistive devices and assistive technology' – emphasises the importance of the philosophy of enabling and promoting self-care, integrated care, self-management and independence. Users of this standard will need to ensure that practice reflects up-to-date information and policies.

To monitor the elderly with chronic conditions in their own residence, telemedicine can be used as a cost-effective way to reduce unnecessary hospitalisation and to ensure that patients receive urgent care in a timely fashion. Telemedicine is used in a more restrictive sense at home and involves the use of technology to monitor the patient's status at a distance.

Studies report that the experience of social isolation in older people has increased and clearly has negative effects on older adults' health, wellbeing and quality of life. Sociability plays an important role in protecting people from the experience of psychological distress and in enhancing well-being. Those caught in poor relationships tend to develop and maintain negative perceptions of self, and tend to find life less satisfying.[12]

Engaging people in their own healthcare is a way to improve people's knowledge, enhance people's experience of services, change service use and cost, and positively impact on people's health.

Social connectedness includes living arrangements, size of social networks and engagement in social activities. Perceived social isolation includes perceptions of social support, as well as feelings of loneliness. Finally, increased social connectedness helps to build up 'social capital'.

Notes

1. Teri, L., Logsdon, R.G. and McCurry, S.M. (2008) 'Exercise interventions for dementia and cognitive impairment: the Seattle Protocols.' *J Nutr Health Aging 12*, 6, 391–394.

2. See, for example, https://www.alzheimers.org.uk/download/downloads/id/1742/the_prime_ministers_challenge_on_dementia_annual_report_of_progress.pdf

3. Accessed on 7 November 2017 at www.alzheimers.org.uk/info/20115/making_your_community_more_dementia-friendly/341/how_to_become_a_recognised_dementia-friendly_community

4. Accessed on 7 November 2017 at https://www.alzheimers.org.uk/download/downloads/id/1918/building_dementia_friendly_communities_a_priority_for_eveyone_-_executive_summary.pdf

5. Green, G. and Lakey, L. (2013) 'Building dementia-friendly communities: a priority for everyone.' Alzheimer's Society. Accessed on 7 November 2017 at www.actonalz.org/sites/default/files/documents/Dementia_friendly_communities_full_report.pdf

6. Smith, K., Gee, S., Sharrock, T. and Croucher, M. (2016) 'Developing a dementia-friendly Christchurch: perspectives of people with dementia.' *Australasian Journal on Ageing 35*, 188–192.

7. Alzheimer's Disease International (2016) 'Dementia Friendly Communities: key principles.' Accessed on 7 November 2017 at www.alz.co.uk/adi/pdf/dfc-principles.pdf

8. See www.meetingdem.eu

9. See www.alzheimers.org.uk/download/downloads/id/3423/this_is_me.pdf

10. See www.kingsfund.org.uk/projects/wanless-social-care-review

11. 'With Respect to Old Age: Long Term Care – Rights and Responsibilities.' A Report by the Royal Commission on Long Term Care, 1999.

12. See, for a fuller discussion, Singh. A. and Misra, N. (2009) 'Loneliness, depression and sociability in old age.' *Ind Psychiatry J 18*, 1, 51–55.

9

Families and care partners as partners in dementia care

The significance of family, care partners and social networks in planning and providing care

---

BOX 9.1 NATIONAL OCCUPATIONAL STANDARDS ON SUPPORTING FAMILIES AND CARE PARTNERS

National Occupational Standard SCDHSC0390 – 'Support families in maintaining relationships in their wider social structures and environments' – identifies the requirements when promoting social inclusion through supporting families to maintain relationships within their community.

National Occupational Standard SFHCMC5 – 'Build a partnership between the team, patients and care partners' – is about developing approaches to patient care in which patients and care partners are active, respected participants.

Outcomes such as meaning making, companionship/sustaining, 'couplehood' and fulfilment have been identified as positive aspects associated with the caregiving experience.

Also, care partner-perceived self-efficacy is associated with increased positive aspects of caregiving. Importantly, rewarding appraisals of and satisfaction with caregiving may reduce stress and improve emotional outcomes that can be associated with caring for a family member diagnosed with Alzheimer's disease.

The significant life changes brought about by a diagnosis of dementia begin a transition from a traditional familial relationship between two loved ones (such as spouse or adult child) to that of a care dyad.

As the person in the role of providing care makes the transition to 'care partner', thoughts about what lies ahead can become overwhelming. Care partners often experience stress during this post-diagnosis period due to a lack of information and knowledge about the diagnosis, and formal resources and support.

Thus, while individuals with dementia may be willing and able to state their preferences for future care, and care partners would benefit from this knowledge of their loved one's wishes, these conversations rarely take place.

Discussions about healthcare preferences are often put off until the later stages of the disease when families may be forced to make critical decisions in a crisis or emergency situation (e.g. the care partner suddenly becomes unable to provide care), and often without input from the person receiving care.

Social networks are defined as 'the structural character of social relationships, such as the number of contacts we have or how often we spend time with those people'.[1] Spousal care partners are supported by pre-existing informal social networks, such as adult children, close relatives, friends and neighbours.

Varying network resources might affect both the wellbeing of the care recipient and family members who provide support and care.

Studies that considered families as caregiving networks have identified compositional characteristics (e.g. larger size, higher proportions of kin and female, proximity of members) associated with more hours of care provided and network typologies (e.g. kin network, friend-based, diffuse-ties network) associated with support availability based on varying network compositions.[3] Thus far, network functions specific to caregiving roles have not been adequately researched.

Care partners of people with dementia can themselves have substantial and unique support needs: they are likely to suffer declines in the availability of people to provide informal support over time, and can tend to disengage from their existing social networks as they devote more time to caring as the disease progresses.

The importance of developing partnerships with family members and care partners

---

BOX 9.2 NATIONAL OCCUPATIONAL STANDARDS
ON PARTNERSHIPS WITH CARE PARTNERS

National Occupational Standard SCDHSC0227 – 'Contribute to working in partnership with care partners' – identifies requirements when you contribute to working in partnership with care partners. This includes working with families and care partners to achieve positive goals and enabling them to review the effectiveness of the support they provide.

National Occupational Standard SCDHSC0387 – 'Work in partnership with care partners to support individuals' – identifies requirements when you work in partnership with care partners to support or care for individuals. This includes working with care partners to access resources, services and facilities to meet their own support needs.

National Occupational Standard SCDHSC0426 – 'Empower families, care partners and others to support individuals' – identifies the requirements when working with families, care partners and others to encourage and enable them to support individuals.

The Triangle of Care – Carers Included: A Guide to Best Practice in Acute Mental Health Care was initially developed by carers with the Princess Royal Trust for Carers and the National Mental Health Development Unit (now Carers Trust), seeking to improve carer engagement in acute inpatient services. The Triangle of Care describes a therapeutic alliance between the person using acute services, staff members and care partners that promotes safety, supports recovery and sustains wellbeing.[3]

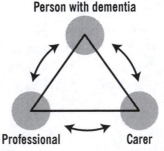

Figure 9.1 The Triangle of Care
Source: Reproduced with permission of Carers Trust from Carers Trust (2016) *The Triangle of Care – Carers Included: A Guide to Best Practice in Acute Mental Health Care.*

It suggests that six key elements are present for care partners when a person receives acute care services:[4]

- Care partners and the essential role they play are identified at first contact or as soon as possible thereafter.

- Staff are 'care partner aware' and trained in care partner engagement strategies.

- Policy and practice protocols about confidentiality and sharing information are in place.

- Defined post(s) responsible for care partners are in place.

- A care partner introduction to the service and staff is available, with a relevant range of information across the acute care pathway.

- A range of care partner support services is available.

The impact that caring for a person with dementia in the family may have on relationships

Caring affects psychological and physical health: the negative health consequences of looking after a family member with dementia are well documented elsewhere. Dementia caregiving has been associated with negative effects on caregiver health, and early nursing home placement for dementia patients.[5] Chronic stress due to caregiving has been linked to poor health outcomes, morbidity and mortality. Preventing and/or ameliorating care partner stress is vital to sustaining family care partners.

But the situation is far more complex than that.

Much of the research has considered the impact upon marital relationships, and less commonly on adult children and their parents or other relationship patterns. Consequently, it is important to view these findings with this in mind, as research considering the experience for the diverse range of relationships, including those influenced by ethnicity, sexual orientation, disability and divorce, is much less in evidence.

Caring for a family member can change family relationships: changes in behaviour and personality can cause family care partners to treat their loved one in a different, more childlike way. Care partners' relationships with siblings can also become strained as the amount of care increases.

Caring full-time can leave family members feeling socially isolated and having to meet hidden costs. And yet caring is often a very rewarding experience that can strengthen family bonds through the close and intimate relationship shared.

The importance of recognising and assessing a care partner's own needs, including respite

BOX 9.3 NATIONAL OCCUPATIONAL STANDARDS ON ASSESSING AND ADDRESSING THE NEEDS OF CARERS

National Occupational Standard SCDHSC0427 – 'Assess the needs of care partners and families' – identifies the requirements when you assess the support needs of care partners and families.

National Occupational Standard SFHCHDHN3 – 'Enable care partners to access and assess support networks and respite services' – is about enabling care partners to access and assess support networks and respite services, ensuring that practice reflects up-to-date information and policies.

A local authority has a duty to assess the care needs of a person with dementia. The assessment will determine what care needs they have, and whether the local authority will contribute towards meeting them. Any person has a right to this assessment, even if they will end up paying for their own care. The process is called a care needs assessment.

The aim is to work out exactly what the person's needs are, and the level and type of care and support required in order to meet these needs. It will also help the local authority to decide whether or not someone is eligible for care and support that will be funded by the council. Even if the person is not eligible, the care needs assessment may still be useful, as it might provide valuable information on the nature and extent of unmet current or future need.

A care needs assessment will usually involve a series of questions, often in the form of a discussion, which the person should be given in advance.

An eligible care need is the level of need that a person must have for the local authority to consider funding it. There are national eligibility criteria that apply across England.

Respite care may take several forms. These range from house-sitting schemes where the care partner is able to take a break of just a few hours, to day care outside the home for a half or whole day, to residential options usually taking the form of regular planned breaks of a few days to several weeks.

Possible reasons for where respite care does not produce benefits include increased workload in preparation for respite care days, the disruption to established routine, guilt, feeling unable to 'let go' while the dependant is receiving respite care, distress at possible deterioration while the dependent is away from home in unfamiliar surroundings and apprehension about his or her return.

In the last decade, there has been a trend towards increased attention to day-care facilities as an important part of community services.

The complexity and diversity in family arrangements

According to the Alzheimer's Society's (2014) 'Dementia: Opportunity for Change',[6] there were approximately 550,000 care partners of people with dementia in England, and family and other informal care partners save the economy approximately £7 billion per year in care costs.

There is marked complexity in family arrangements due to the composition of numerous interconnected, semi-autonomous, competing and collaborating members within the family. The members of a family working as part of a complex adaptive system can be individuals, teams, functional groups, social institutions or organisational processes.

Demographic and social trends influence caregiving in families with older members. The conventional nuclear family model is increasingly uncommon as new, pluralistic models of family life are emerging in contemporary society. The majority of elder care is provided by relatives, albeit with varying patterns of involvement and responsibility across family structures.

Additional research on family risk and resilience related to the care of older relatives is warranted, particularly with respect to pluralistic models of family life.

The needs of care partners and the person with dementia may not always be the same

As dementia progresses, the needs of both the person with dementia and their care partner are likely to change significantly, and at some point it may become appropriate for the person to move into residential care, or for more formal support to be provided in the person's own home.

It is imperative in such circumstances that the care partner's continuing role is acknowledged, and that care partners should be given opportunities to sustain whatever input they are able to contribute to the care for as long as they wish.

Some care partners will wish to continue providing particular forms of care and support, such as washing their loved one's clothes or taking in favourite food, even where the person with dementia is being cared for in a residential environment.

Potential sociocultural differences in the perception of the caregiving role

Numerous studies have shown that caring for an older family member with chronic health problems and functional limitations is associated with more negative mental and physical health outcomes.

Greater theoretical and methodological precision regarding the examination of caregiving across different ethnic and cultural groups will help to inform the content of interventions and services aimed at alleviating care partners' distress among individuals from diverse backgrounds.

Literature reviews on ethnicity and caregiving have emphasised the need to explicitly measure and assess the impact that cultural values have on caregiving experiences instead of simply using group membership to examine cultural and ethnic differences in caregiving.

The impact on younger care partners and their concerns

Most studies of care partners of persons with dementia do not separate spouses or cohabitants from adult children.

Many young adult care partners aged between 16 and 18 years are at increased risk of not being in education, employment or training, and report that they have mental health problems.

Dementia develops gradually and the family might encounter challenges. Many services are only funded to work with young care partners up to the age of 18. In a survey, 79 per cent of young care partners overall said they were worried about moving on as they felt there was no support for them.[7]

The patient's memory impairment might make it difficult to remember appointments and messages; therefore, foresight and planning in the family are disturbed. The children can become worried, confused and fearful when important information is forgotten.

Some children and adolescents experience guilt and shame, and feel embarrassed when their friends meet their parent who is forgetful or exhibits a change in personality.

The need to communicate compassionately, effectively and in a timely manner with care partners

Individual differences such as attachment style and marital satisfaction also affect how care partners perceive and respond emotionally to a partner's emotional state.

For example, care partners who are more anxiously attached (i.e. worry about receiving care and love from others) experience more feelings of personal distress compared with care partners who are less anxiously attached. In contrast, care partners who have more avoidant attachments (i.e. they are uncomfortable with intimacy and dependence on others) report feeling less personal distress.

Compassion is one of 'the 6Cs'.[8] Care, compassion, courage, communication, commitment and competence are a central plank of Compassion in Practice, introduced by NHS England. The values and behaviours covered by the 6Cs are not, in themselves, a new concept. However, putting them together in this way to define a vision is an opportunity in strategic policy to reinforce the enduring values and beliefs that underpin care wherever it takes place.

The need to support family care partners to access and use information and local support networks

After receiving the diagnosis, specific information is needed to provide a better understanding of the disease. This could help with care planning and offer some relief of tension within the family.

The diagnosis is often a source of uncertainty as people struggle to find any explanations within the healthcare system. This elicits feelings of anxiety and helplessness, and as a consequence, care partners have often searched for information themselves.

Care partners often report that they would have liked to receive information on the type of help available, especially in the period immediately after they are given the diagnosis.

In addition, they describe a wish to learn more about the disease and treatment options, and to talk about practical issues such as adapting their home, how to provide specific care, whom to contact in case of emergencies and where to obtain help with financial issues.

Care partners worry about the course of the illness and the possibility of upcoming institutionalisation.

The need to support family care partners in considering options and making decisions

Shared decision-making is a consultative process where a clinician and patient jointly participate in making a health decision, having discussed the options and their benefits and harms, and having considered the patient's values, preferences and circumstances.

Shared decision-making is not a single step to be added into a consultation, but can provide a framework for communicating with patients about healthcare choices to help improve conversation quality.

The need to gather information about a person's history and preferences from family care partners

Caring for the whole person requires professionals to engage with people receiving care as individuals with a collection of problems, preferences and needs – including other health conditions, social issues and wider circumstances – rather than narrowly focusing on a particular task or condition.

The nature of contemporary care facilitates a 'whole-person approach' – visiting people in their own homes helps staff to gather critical information about the wellbeing, needs and preferences of the person through seeing them in their home environment and speaking to formal and informal care partners and family.

Contributing to the development of practices and services that meet the needs of families and care partners

BOX 9.4 NATIONAL OCCUPATIONAL STANDARDS ON DEVELOPING PROGRAMMES TO SUPPORT CARERS AND FAMILIES

National Occupational Standard SCDHSC0428 – 'Lead the development of programmes of support for care partners and families' – identifies the requirements when you lead on developing programmes of support for care partners and families of individuals who use health and social care services.

Understanding methods to assess a care partner's psychological and practical needs and the relevant support available

Many people with dementia, with met and unmet needs, receive help from a family member or friend. It is estimated that three-quarters of older people with moderate to severe dementia living in the community have a family care partner. Looking after another person affects people's lives in many and various ways. Support to care partners needs to reflect such individual differences.

Many care partners report difficulties in having their needs met. Practical help with day-to-day situations makes a positive difference to care partners' lives.

Individuals respond to caring in different ways, so help needs to vary accordingly. A single service is unlikely to meet care partners' ongoing needs fully; diverse preferences require a wide range of services.

Care partners appreciate assessments which result in good access to information, potential access to a new or additional service and the opportunity to discuss their circumstances in an objective way.

Care partners feel it is important to be included in decision-making, have their expertise valued, know whom to contact if needed and have a service that is responsive to their needs. They are also pivotal in acute admissions of persons with dementia to hospital. The impact of John's Campaign[9] has been striking here.

Understanding the potential for dilemmas arising where there are differing needs between people with dementia and their care partners

With increasing severity of dementia, decision-making capacity decreases. This is a threat to autonomy and persons with dementia need help to compensate for declining abilities.

In dementia care, as in *all* healthcare, the principle of beneficence is the primary obligation. It entails a moral obligation to act for the benefit of others and prevent harm. Non-maleficence, on the other hand, means not inflicting harm.

Paternalism has been conceptualised as the opposite of autonomy and can be defined as:

> ...the intentional overriding of one person's preferences or actions by another person, where the person who overrides justifies this action by appeal to the goal of benefitting or of preventing or mitigating harm to the person whose preferences or actions are overridden.[10]

Paternalism is thus a relevant issue in dementia care and may involve soft paternalism where helpers interfere by gently persuading or acting in such a manner that they do not let persons make poor choices or they protect them against the potentially harmful consequences of their own stated preferences or actions.

The question of autonomy in dementia care is especially challenging in light of how vulnerable people with dementia are when living at home. They are perceived to be at risk for problems with nutrition, falls, personal hygiene, drug management, fire hazards, getting lost, financial fraud and social isolation. These risks threaten autonomy.

Caring for people with dementia living at home can create ethical dilemmas of how to balance autonomy with their safety and wellbeing. A dilemma can be defined as '(a) a difficult problem seemingly incapable of a satisfactory solution or (b) a situation involving choice between equally unsatisfactory alternatives. An ethical dilemma arises when values and moral positions or claims conflict with one another.'[11]

A recent study found that professional care partners could sometimes trivialise older people's complaints and only allowed them to influence their daily activities if this did not conflict with procedures in the institution.[12]

Understanding the role of personalisation in care (e.g. the impact of access to personal budgets)

Personalisation means recognising people as individuals who have strengths and preferences and putting them at the centre of their own care and support. The traditional service-led approach has often meant that people have not been able to shape the kind of support they need or receive the right kind of help.

Personalised approaches such as self-directed support and personal budgets involve enabling people to identify their own needs and make choices about how and when they are supported to live their lives. People need access to information, advocacy and advice so they can make informed decisions.

Personalisation is a relatively new term and there are different ideas about what it could mean and how it will work in practice. Personalisation might mean:

- tailoring support to people's individual needs whatever the care and support setting

- using 'co-production' to support people to actively engage in the design, delivery and evaluation of services

- recognising and supporting care partners in their role, while enabling them to maintain a life beyond their caring responsibilities

- ensuring all citizens have access to universal community services and resources.

The Department of Health makes it clear that, importantly, the ability to make choices about how people live their lives should not be restricted only to those who live in their own homes.[13] It is about better support, more tailored to individual choices, and preferences in all care settings.

This must have at least equal resonance for those living in residential care homes and other institutions, where personalised approaches may be less developed. Here, the independent sector has a crucial role to play in delivering personalised solutions for people no longer living in their own homes.

Rather than fitting the person to services, services should fit the person.

Person-centred care has the same meaning as person-centred planning, but is more commonly used in the field of dementia care and services for older people.

Notes

1. Soulsby, L.K. and Bennett, K.M. (2015) 'How relationships help us to age well.' *The Psychologist* *28*, 2, 110–113.
2. Koehly, L.M., Ashida, S., Schafer, E.J. and Ludden, A. (2015) 'Caregiving networks-using a network approach to identify missed opportunities.' *J Gerontol B Psychol Sci Soc Sci 70*, 1, 143–154.
3. Accessed on 4 October 2017 at https://professionals.carers.org/sites/default/files/thetriangleofcare_guidetobestpracticeinmentalhealthcare_england.pdf
4. Carers Trust (2016) *The Triangle of Care – Carers Included: A Guide to Best Practice in Acute Mental Health Care*, p.3.
5. See, for example, Etters, L., Goodall, D. and Harrison, B.E. (2008) 'Caregiver burden among dementia patient caregivers: a review of the literature.' *J Am Acad Nurse Pract 20*, 8, 423–428.
6. Accessed on 4 October 2017 at www.alzheimers.org.uk/download/downloads/id/2317/dementia_2014_opportunity_for_change.pdf
7. See https://care partners.org/key-facts-about-care partners-and-people-they-care
8. NHS England, 'The 6Cs.' Accessed on 4 October 2017 at www.england.nhs.uk/leadingchange/about/the-6cs
9. See http://johnscampaign.org.uk
10. Beauchamp, T.L. and Childress, J.F. (2012) *Principles of Biomedical Ethics 7*. Oxford: Oxford University Press, p.215.
11. Davies, A.J., Fowler, M.D. and Aroskar, M.A. (2010) *Ethical Dilemmas and Nursing Practice*. New York: Pearson Prentice Hall, p.7.
12. Persson, T. and Wästerfors, D. (2009) '"Such trivial matters": How staff account for restrictions of residents' influence in nursing homes.' *Journal of Aging Studies 23*, 1, 1–11.
13. See, for example, King's Fund (2010) 'People in control of their own health and care: The state of involvement.' Accessed on 7 November 2017 at www.kingsfund.org.uk/sites/default/files/field/field_publication_file/people-in-control-of-their-own-health-and-care-the-state-of-involvement-november-2014.pdf

10

Equality, diversity and inclusion in dementia care

Cultural diversity and equality issues, and how they may impact on people with dementia

You can reduce the chances of discrimination happening by the way you work. As a health or social care worker, it is your duty to work in ways that promote:

- equality

- diversity

- inclusion.

These principles should be included into everything that you do. To achieve this, you should:

- respect diversity by providing person-centred care

- treat the individuals you support as unique rather than treating all individuals in the same way

- work in an inclusive way that sees the positive input that all individuals can make to society and to their own care

- be confident to challenge or confront any discriminatory practice if you see this in your workplace.

Inclusion is a human right for every individual. The aim of inclusion is to embrace all people irrespective of race, gender, disability, medical or other need, culture, age, religion and sexual orientation. It is about giving equal access and opportunities and getting rid of discrimination and intolerance.

Inclusion is recognising our universal 'oneness' and interdependence. Inclusion is recognising that we are *one* even though we are not the *same*.

The act of inclusion means fighting against exclusion. Fighting for inclusion involves making sure that all support systems are available to those who need support. It is everyone's responsibility to remove the barriers to inclusion.

Support and care services should be delivered in a culturally appropriate manner, for example:

- meeting a person's dietary requirements

- speaking a person's language

- creating an environment in which people could express their religious views and celebrate religious occasions.

Studies also reveal various interpretations of dementia across different cultures and acknowledge the importance of considering such variations when diagnosing dementia. One ethnographic study revealed that clinicians who consider religion and culture when making a diagnosis of dementia can develop a different interpretation of symptoms they might otherwise consider to be symptomatic of dementia.[1]

A key aspect of caregiving that is seen in many cultures is the central role of the family.

The Spanish concept of *familismo* means that the needs of the family are prioritised over the needs of individuals within the family; this influences families' decisions about providing care.

Age

The Equality and Human Rights Commission has uncovered serious, systemic threats to the basic human rights of older people who are getting home care services.

Their findings suggest that age discrimination is one of the key factors explaining why older people face risks to their human rights in home care services.[2] They have also uncovered examples of where someone's age determines the funding and provision of home care services.

The challenges for unpaid care partners of someone with dementia are well documented, but arguably the situations of those caring for someone with young-onset dementia are particularly difficult because of its timing.

The age of people with young-onset dementia means that the symptoms of dementia may lead to loss of employment. The implications of unemployment are manifold and include financial, psychological and social consequences, such as changed or difficult family relationships, poor self-esteem and reduced sense of competency and purpose.

Disability

The definition of disability in the Equality Act 2010 also includes dementia.

In March 2013, there were approximately 462,910 places in care homes in England according to the Care Quality Commission (CQC).[3] According to the CQC report:

- A large number of people using regulated social care services would be protected by disability discrimination law – even if many of them (particularly older people) do not self-identify as disabled.

- Approximately 278,000 care home places have been identified as being for people with dementia.

- Among people living in care homes, hospital admissions for avoidable conditions were 30 per cent higher for those who had dementia compared with those without dementia.[4]

Disabled people under 65 may use social care for long periods – even for the whole of their lives, whether they have a physical or sensory impairment, a learning disability or use mental health services.

The way that social care is organised and delivered can be a critical factor in disabled citizens being able to exercise their human rights over a large proportion of their adult lives. Independence is a fundamental human rights principle which underpins other human rights.

The Joint Committee on Human Rights report on the rights of disabled people to independent living reaffirms the importance of independent-living principles for all disabled people, including those in residential care.[5]

Disabled people have rights to independent living enshrined in Article 19 of the United Nations Convention on the Rights of People with Disabilities (UNCRPD), to which the UK is a signatory. The report makes a number of recommendations about upholding these rights including the role of regulation in this.

Ethnicity

People from all ethnic groups are affected by dementia. The number of people with dementia in minority ethnic groups has been estimated to be around 15,000 in England, and there may be a lower degree of knowledge of dementia among some ethnic groups.[6]

There is an issue as to whether current services for people with dementia and their family care partners adequately take account of cultural differences both in terms of timely diagnosis and post-diagnostic care and support.

Ethnicity can be a significant factor in the extent to which dementia is understood or acknowledged, or in people's willingness to seek help.

There is substantial evidence about the increasing numbers of people with dementia, of the growing population of older people from black, Asian and minority ethnic (BAME) groups in the UK and the need to enable ageing in place (that is, living in the residence of their choice, for as long as they are able, as they age) among older people with or without dementia where possible and desired.

The number of people with dementia from BAME groups is expected to rise significantly as the BAME population ages. The Centre for Policy on Ageing and the Runnymede Trust estimate that there are nearly 25,000 people with dementia from BAME communities in England and Wales, a number that is expected to grow to almost 50,000 by 2026 and more than 172,000 by 2051.[7]

Religion and belief

There are many ways in which religion and beliefs have an impact on social care provision, such as:

- diet, including the type of food that can or cannot be eaten

- fasting times observed by some religions – for example, Hindus and Muslims

- Orthodox Jews' observance of the Sabbath.

Adaptation of assessment and care planning taking account of equality issues (e.g. cultural diversity, disabilities, gender and sexual orientation)

Each person is treated as an individual and care services are responsive to his or her race, culture, religion, age, disability, gender (including gender identity) and sexual orientation.

People can take part in activities that are appropriate to their age and culture, and are part of their local community. They are able to keep in touch with family, friends and representatives, and they are supported to have appropriate personal, family and sexual relationships.

People are as independent as they can be, lead their chosen lifestyle and have the opportunity to make the most of their abilities. Their dignity and rights are respected in their daily life.

Age discrimination is an additional factor since dementia is an illness of later life, and age discrimination accentuates the role of stigma. This has been called 'double jeopardy'. It is this facet of awareness and diagnosis where women may suffer greater disadvantage than their male counterparts.

Age discrimination against women is well documented in many societies and therefore it seems that older women affected by conditions such as dementia are exposed to what we could term a 'triple jeopardy' – discriminated against as a result of their age, gender and condition.

Women and dementia

There is, as figures and projections show, a near-universal gender gap in life expectancy in favour of women.

Women are more likely to live in communal establishments (including care homes) with some exceptions in different ethnic groups.[8] There are a number of reasons that may contribute to this difference, including the differing age profile of men and women, which increases with age. This difference, and the fact that the social care workforce is predominantly female, can mean that it is harder to meet the gender-specific needs of men in care homes.

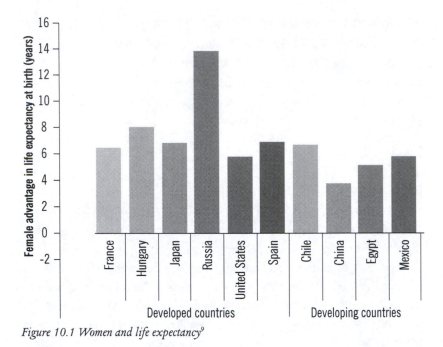

Figure 10.1 Women and life expectancy[9]

Generally speaking, the majority of people affected by dementia are women. It is estimated that 61 per cent of people with dementia are women and 39 per cent are men.[10] This is likely to be because women live longer than men, as age is the biggest known risk factor for the condition.[11]

However, different dementia subtypes may have different prevalent rates and so life expectancy is not the only factor to consider. In addition to there being a greater prevalence of dementia amongst women than men, a greater proportion of caregivers are women, reported by a number of studies to be between 60–70 per cent.[12]

Care partners are thus arguably a forgotten and invisible workforce and are overlooked in terms of health and social care support. Unpaid care partners provide a prop for ailing health and social care systems in the developed world and remain the bedrock of most forms of elder care in the developing world.

Because age is the single biggest risk factor, the majority of people living with dementia are also older, aged 65 years and above. Thus, it is important to consider gender in the context of ageing when discussing this topic.

There is also the wider issue pertaining to gender bias against women in several areas of clinical research. Women historically were excluded from early studies of most drug trials due to reasons of safety. This gender bias in research may have potential repercussions for evidence-based medicine and the future disease management of dementia syndromes.

Gender and sexual orientation

Commissioners and providers of social care and healthcare often fail to consider the needs of lesbian, gay, bisexual, transsexual or transgender and intersex (LGBTI) people when planning and/or running services.

Assuming that all people are heterosexual or cisgender, they may unwittingly discriminate against those who are not heterosexual or who do not identify with the gender they were assigned at birth.

Often LGBTI people feel services will not meet their needs or be sensitive to them, and people who are LBGTI with dementia may not have previously identified as being LGBTI due to having been inhibited as a result of stigma or discrimination. It is not known how many LGBTI people are currently living in care homes or hospices.

Kitwood[13] characterises 'personhood' as the specific attributes an individual possesses that make them a person. He uses this term in a theory of dementia care that advocates maintaining the personhood of people with dementia through appreciating their unique biopsychosocial circumstances, including their sexuality. Important psychological components of personhood include safety and comfort, inclusion, occupation and a valued identity.

Research is needed to assess how personhood is maintained for LGBTI individuals whose sexuality may be obscured by their diagnosis, as person-centred dementia care involves the acknowledgement of sexual orientation.

Within residential settings, older LGBTI individuals have identified that care staff, administration staff and other residents can all be sources of discrimination. In these contexts, within which institutional homophobia or perceived discrimination is encountered, psychological safety in relation to personhood may be under threat.

Diversity in family arrangements and the local community

BOX 10.1 DIVERSITY IN FAMILIES[14]

In 2011 there were an estimated 17.9 million families in the UK, an increase from 17.0 million in 2001, with the increase of 0.7 million cohabiting couple families and 0.4 million lone parent families offset by a decrease of 0.3 million in the number of married couple families.

There were an estimated 50.7 million people living in families in the UK in 2011, an increase from 48.8 million in 2001.

The most common type of family in the UK in 2010 was a married couple with or without children, although the proportion had decreased from an estimated 72.4 per cent of all families in 2001 to 67.2 per cent in 2011.

In the UK families consisting of a cohabiting couple with or without children increased from 12.5 per cent of all families in 2001 to 16.0 per cent 2011, and lone parent families increased from 14.8 per cent in 2001 to 16.1 per cent in 2011.

The most common type of family with children in the UK contained one child at the time of the survey in 2011 (46.3 per cent of all families with children).

The shift from a high-mortality/high-fertility society to a low-mortality/low-fertility society results in an increase in the number of living generations, and a decrease in the number of living relatives within these generations.

Within the white majority population of the UK, we are seeing the emergence of long vertical multigenerational families replacing the former laterally extended family forms. Increased longevity may increase the duration spent in certain kinship roles, such as spouse, parent of non-dependent child, sibling.

A decrease in fertility may reduce the duration of others, such as parent of dependent child, or even the opportunity for some roles, such as sibling. Changing family structures may well be different for BAME groups and the lesbian, gay, bisexual and transgender communities.

Of the 7.7 million one-person households in the UK, 54.2 per cent of them in 2016 contained one woman and 45.8 per cent of them contained one man.[15]

Stigma, myths and stereotypes associated with dementia

Attention to the rights, dignity and wellbeing of people with dementia has increased in recent years. There has been an increased interest in developing dementia-friendly communities and other initiatives, the development of national dementia strategies throughout Europe, and the 'Glasgow Declaration', which calls on the European Commission to develop a European dementia strategy.

However, dementia is still often perceived as a stigma.

Stigma is a complex social phenomenon involving a process whereby people sharing a socially salient group difference are identified and subsequently devalued and discriminated against, either overtly or covertly. This may be accompanied by a private process whereby the stigmatised person or group internalises the perceived stigmatising attitudes of others.

Stigma is also the term used to refer to the attribute, which is discrediting, in that it reduces someone in other people's minds from a 'whole and usual person to a tainted, discounted one'.[16] The attribute is not stigmatising in itself but may become so depending on the meanings people attach to it (i.e. it is socially constructed).

Consequently, although there is a general agreement about the need to challenge the stigma of dementia, we need to understand better the meanings associated with dementia which contribute towards it being perceived as a stigma.

In addition to the social and emotional impact of the perception of dementia as a stigma, there are also implications for health in that the stigma of dementia has been linked to delays in timely diagnosis.

Relatively little is known about the meanings that medical professionals associate with dementia or what they believe the general public associate with dementia, but the opinions and perceptions of healthcare professionals may be similar in some ways to those of the general public.

If general practitioners' understanding of the way that dementia is perceived as a stigma in society was similar to that of the general public, and this overshadowed their medical knowledge, training and expertise, they would be ill-placed to play a role in helping tackle such stigma.

Stigma has been seen as including three aspects, namely stereotypes, prejudice and discrimination.

Stereotypes describe collective judgements about groups of people (e.g. people with dementia); prejudice refers to emotional reactions to a stereotyped person; and discrimination refers to behaviours that are associated with prejudice, including avoidance, coercion and segregation.

Prevalence and impact of young-onset dementia

Young-onset dementia refers to dementia that happens before the age of 65.

The Alzheimer's Society estimates there are approximately 42,000 younger people with dementia in the UK. This equates to 5 per cent of all people with dementia. This is an important consideration for organisations providing care and support services.

Until about 20 years ago, medical professionals and the public assumed that dementia mainly affected people over the age of 65, and this is perhaps why research is usually focused on this age group.

There are currently no national studies of the number of people with young-onset dementia because such studies depend on a large number of people taking part to produce an accurate estimate of that number.

There are only a handful of local studies on the prevalence of young-onset dementia, one being a study on three London boroughs in 2003. This found that the prevalence rate of young-onset dementia in those aged between 30 and 64 was 54 per 100,000 people; and in the 45–64 age group it was 98 per 100,000 people.[17]

Legislation to support care partners, including young care partners

The 2011 Census revealed that there were more than 1.8 million care partners aged 60 and over in England – almost 16 per cent of the population of this age range. This includes a huge 20 per cent of the population in the 60–64 age group, compared with 12.6 per cent of the overall population. The number of care partners aged 85 and over grew by 128 per cent over the last decade.[18]

This group is often invisible, with many older care partners providing long hours of vital care and support while their own health and wellbeing deteriorates, resulting in poor physical and mental health, financial strain and breakdown in their ability to carry on caring.

A care partner is someone who helps another person, usually a relative or friend, in their day-to-day life. This is not the same as someone who provides care professionally or through a voluntary organisation.

The Care Act 2014 sets out care partners' legal rights to assessment and support. It came into force in April 2015. The Care Act relates mostly to adult care partners – people aged 18 and over who are caring for another adult. This is because young care partners (aged under 18) and adults who care for disabled children can be assessed and supported under children's law.

The Care Act gives local authorities a responsibility to assess a care partner's need for support, where the care partner appears to have such needs. This replaced the law that required that the care partner had to be providing 'a substantial amount of care on a regular basis' to qualify for an assessment. This means more care partners are now able to have an assessment. The care partner will be entitled to support if they are assessed as having needs that meet the eligibility criteria and the person they care for lives in the local authority area (which means their established home is in that local authority area).

The Children and Families Act 2014 is an important new piece of legislation for young care partners, young adult care partners and their families. It amends Section 17 of the Children Act 1989.

Young care partners, young adult care partners and their families now have stronger rights to be identified, offered information, receive an assessment and be supported using a whole-family approach.

Local authorities must meet their duties to identify, assess and support young care partners, young adult care partners and their families. They will need to work with other local organisations to make sure they are proactively identifying all young care partners.

Additional concerns of younger care partners

Service provision has tended to focus on the person living with dementia and their primary care partners.

However, many of the young people living with a parent with young-onset dementia can have emotional problems themselves, problems at school and conflict with the parent with young-onset dementia, said to be more common if the father is affected.

Moreover, these young people can feel isolated and are often ill-equipped for the caring role they find themselves in.

A recent report looking at caring responsibilities of young care partners across a broad range of situations, not specific to young-onset dementia, has emphasised the association with young care partners' mental and physical health and its deterioration over time, particularly as young care partners move into adulthood.[19]

Typically, shame of their parents' behaviour caused social isolation – for example, where friends were not invited to their house, which further affected their relationship with their parent. The distress associated with living with a parent with young-onset dementia needs to be seen in the context of the health and wellbeing of the broader population of young people.

In addition to the lack of research on the impacts on young people of living with a parent with young-onset dementia, there is little guidance in the literature around service needs of these young people.

Young people are affected in many ways when a parent develops a disability, whether it is physical or psychological, and there is often significant financial hardship. In many families, the other parent has to take on more paid work as well as the dual role of caring for their partner and family, which can often lead to the affected young people going unnoticed.

The impact of dementia on people with learning disabilities

Dementia may be more common in older adults with intellectual disability than in the general population. In one study it is argued that the incidence of dementia in older people with intellectual disabilities is up to five times higher than older adults in the general population.[20]

Dementia often presents differently in adults with intellectual disability and varies depending on the nature and severity of intellectual disability.

In Down's syndrome, changes reflective of frontal lobe dysfunction (personality, emotion and behaviour changes) are often noted before changes in language ability or memory.

In non-Down's syndrome intellectual disability, the most common early sign of dementia reported by care partners is general deterioration, followed by emotional and behavioural change.

Premature onset of other medical co-morbidities could also affect cognitive function.

In addition to physical co-morbidities, life events (such as bereavement) or changes in an individual's circumstances (change in residence or staff members) could result in a decline in behaviour and cognition that is incorrectly attributed to dementia.

Some key points are provided in 'Dementia and People with Intellectual Disabilities',[21] including that:

people with intellectual disabilities, their families and care partners need to be given opportunities to understand the nature of the intellectual disability and information about any associated health risks from an early point in their life and particularly from transition to adulthood onwards.

Challenging any discriminatory practice that may compromise a person's right to dignity and respect

Discrimination is a preconceived attitude towards members of a particular group formed only upon the basis of their membership of that group that leads to less favourable or bad treatment of that person. The attitude is often resistant to change even in the light of new information.

It is essential that prejudices are not allowed to influence the way professionals and practitioners work with individuals.

Most people have experienced discrimination in one way or another. Some people are more likely to suffer discrimination. These people might be older people, young people, females, disabled people, homosexuals, lesbians, transgender people and members of ethnic minorities.

Discrimination is action that is often based on a person's negative attitude towards others. It involves treating people differently because of assumptions made about a person or group of people based on their differences.

Negative attitudes and behaviours exist in society that can lead to individuals or groups being oppressed or disadvantaged.

BOX 10.2 NATIONAL OCCUPATIONAL STANDARDS ON UPHOLDING THE RIGHTS OF INDIVIDUALS

National Occupational Standard SCDHSC0234 – 'Uphold the rights of individuals' – identifies the requirements when you uphold the rights of individuals. This includes upholding individuals' right to be in control of their lives, to be respected for who they are, and to have information about themselves kept private.

National Occupational Standard SCDHSC0452 – 'Lead practice that promotes the rights, responsibilities, equality and diversity' – identifies the requirements when you lead practice to promote the rights, responsibilities, equality and diversity of individuals. This includes leading practice to ensure that systems promote individuals' rights and respect diversity.

National Occupational Standard SCDHSC3111 – 'Promote the rights and diversity of individuals' – identifies the requirements when you promote the rights and diversity of individuals. This includes promoting a culture that values and respects the diversity of all individuals.

National Occupational Standard SFHSS01 – 'Foster people's equality, diversity and rights' – is about acknowledging the equality and diversity of people, their rights and responsibilities.

International human rights law

In addition to the Universal Declaration of Human Rights (UDHR) are the UN human rights treaties that are at the core of the international system for the promotion and protection of human rights.

Every UN member state is a party to one or more of the nine major human rights treaties. Together these form a universal and inalienable human rights system which applies to every child, woman or man in the world. The UK has ratified a number of the UN's international human rights conventions, including the UN Convention on the Rights of Persons with Disabilities and its Optional Protocol 2008.

The European Convention on Human Rights and European Court on Human Rights

The Council of Europe gave effect to the UDHR through the European Convention on Human Rights (ECHR) which was signed in 1950 and ratified by the United Kingdom in 1951. The Council of Europe now comprises 47 member countries, all of which subscribe to the ECHR. The Convention is divided into Articles, and Articles 2 to 14 set out the rights that are protected by the Convention.

(The European Court of Human Rights (ECtHR) is not to be confused with the European Court of Justice (ECJ) which is based in Luxembourg and is the highest court of the European Union in matters of European Community law, but not national law.)

The impact that discrimination and stigma may have on the life of the person with dementia, their family and care partners

Despite UK government imperatives designed to reduce discriminatory practice, there remain a number of ambiguities that will continue to affect professionals' positive attitude formation towards this client group.

Inequity of funding for older people's mental health services will continue to undermine efforts to develop practice and services for people with dementia, and with that the climate of professional socialisation.

It is essential that greater emphasis on self-awareness and anti-discriminatory practice is integrated into nursing curricula; otherwise, it is unlikely that real change will occur at the level of direct care in the near future.

Overall discrimination experiences of care partners, which can have an effect upon their health, include:

- no time to eat properly

- physical and mental exhaustion

- difficulty in doing your own job.

Social care services have the potential to have a large positive impact on the lives of people providing unpaid care.

Legislation relevant to equality, diversity and human rights

The Equality Act 2010 made it unlawful for people to be treated unfairly because of the things that make them different. The Act sets out how individuals should experience equality of opportunity and lists a number of 'protected characteristics' that help to safeguard them from discrimination.

The Act has the aim of promoting equality and respecting diversity to help to ensure that people are valued and have the same access to all opportunities whatever their differences.

Protected characteristics, stated in the Act, aim to protect these groups of individuals from experiencing discrimination. The nine protected characteristics are:

- age

- disability

- gender reassignment

- marriage and civil partnership

- pregnancy and maternity

- race

- religion or belief

- sex

- sexual orientation.

The Human Rights Act 1998 incorporates the Articles of the ECHR into UK law. It did not create any new rights but made it clear that as far as possible the courts in this country should interpret the law in a way that is compatible with the Convention rights.

The Act sets out the ways in which everyone should be treated by the state and by public authorities. It also places an obligation on public authorities to act compatibly with Convention rights. If an Act of Parliament breaches these Convention rights, the courts can declare the legislation to be incompatible.

The Mental Capacity Act 2005 is designed to protect people who can't make decisions for themselves.

The Care Act 2014 brings care and support legislation together into a single act with a new wellbeing principle at its heart. It aims to make care and support clearer and fairer and to put people's wellbeing at the centre of decisions, and include and develop personalisation.

The Health and Social Care Act 2012 set out to 'modernise' NHS care by supporting new services and giving patients a greater voice in their care.

Notes

1. Elliot, K.S., and Di Minno, M. (2006) 'Unruly grandmothers, ghosts and ancestors: Chinese elders and the importance of culture in dementia evaluations.' *Journal of Cross Cultural Gerontology* 21, 157–177.
2. EHRC (2011) 'Close to Home: An inquiry into older people and human rights in home care.' Accessed on 7 November 2017 at www.equalityhumanrights.com/sites/default/files/close_to_home.pdf
3. Care Quality Commission (2014) 'Equality counts: Equality information for CQC in 2013.' Accessed on 4 October 2017 at www.cqc.org.uk/sites/default/files/documents/edhr_annual_report_january_2014final.pdf
4. Care Quality Commission (2013) 'The state of health care and adult social care in England in 2012/13.' Accessed on 4 October 2017 at www.cqc.org.uk/sites/default/files/documents/cqc_soc_report_2013_lores2.pdf

5. Joint Committee on Human Rights (2012) 'Implementation of the Right of Disabled People to Independent Living.' Accessed on 4 October 2017 at www.publications.parliament.uk/pa/jt201012/jtselect/jtrights/257/257.pdf

6. Healthcare for London (2011) Dementia Services Guide, Appendix 9: Equality Impact Assessment. Accessed on 4 October 2017 at www.londonhp.nhs.uk/wp-content/uploads/2011/03/09-Dementia-EqIA.pdf

7. Cited in All-Party Parliamentary Group on Dementia (2013) 'Dementia does not discriminate: The experience of black, Asian and minority ethnic communities.' Accessed on 4 October 2017 at www.alzheimers.org.uk/download/downloads/id/1857/appg_2013_bame_report.pdf

8. Care Quality Commission (2014) 'Equality counts: Equality information for CQC in 2013. Accessed on 4 October 2017 at www.cqc.org.uk/sites/default/files/documents/edhr_annual_report_january_2014final.pdf

9. Adapted from Figure 2 'Females Advantage in Life Expectancy at Birth for Selected Countries in 2008' (Obtained from the US Census Bureau Database)' in Bamford, S.-M. (2011) 'Women and Dementia – Not forgotten', p.16, The International Longevity Centre UK (ILC-UK). Accessed on 4 October 2017 at www.mscforum.pt/images/Women_and_Dementia_pdf_191.pdf

10. Alzheimer's Research UK (2015) 'Women and Dementia: A Marginalised Majority.' Accessed on 4 October 2017 at www.alzheimersresearchuk.org/wp-content/uploads/2015/03/Women-and-Dementia-A-Marginalised-Majority1.pdf

11. Alzheimer's Disease International (2015) 'Women and Dementia: A global research review.' Accessed on 4 October at www.alz.co.uk/sites/default/files/pdfs/Women-and-Dementia.pdf

12. Alzheimer's Disease International (2015) 'Women and Dementia: A global research review.' Accessed on 7 November 2017 at www.alz.co.uk/sites/default/files/pdfs/Women-and-Dementia.pdf

13. Kitwood, T. (1997) *Dementia Reconsidered: The Person Comes First.* Buckingham: Open University Press.

14. From Macrory, I./Office for National Statistics (2012) 'Measuring National Well-being – Households and Families, 2012'. Accessed on 4 October at http://webarchive.nationalarchives.gov.uk/20160105160709/http://www.ons.gov.uk/ons/dcp171766_259965.pdf

15. Office for National Statistics (2016) 'Families and households in the UK: 2016.' Accessed on 4 October at www.ons.gov.uk/peoplepopulationandcommunity/birthsdeathsandmarriages/families/bulletins/familiesandhouseholds/2016

16. Goffman, E. (1963) *Stigma.* London: Penguin.

17. Social Care Institute for Excellence (2013) 'Dementia Gateway: Young Onset Dementia.' Accessed on 4 October 2017 at www.scie.org.uk/dementia/resources/files/young-onset-dementia.pdf

18. Carers UK and Age UK (2015) 'Caring into later life: The growing pressure on older carers.' Accessed on 4 October 2017 at www.carersuk.org/for-professionals/policy/policy-library/caring-into-later-life

19. Cass, B., Brennan, D., Thomson, C., Hill, T. *et al.* (2011) 'Young carers: Social policy impacts of the caring responsibilities of children and young adults.' Report prepared for ARC Linkage Partners, October 2011. Accessed on 4 October 2017 at www.adhc.nsw.gov.au/__data/assets/file/0005/255686/Young_Carers_Report_Final_October_2011_w_cover_page.pdf

20. Strydom, A., Chan, T., King, M., Hassiotis, A. and Livingston, G. (2013) 'Incidence of dementia in older adults with intellectual disabilities.' Res Dev Disabil. 2013 Jun;34(6):1881-5. doi: 10.1016/j.ridd.2013.02.021. Epub 2013 Apr 9. http://www.sciencedirect.com/science/article/pii/S0891422213000851?via%3Dihub

21. Faculty for People with Intellectual Disabilities of the British Psychological Society Division of Clinical Psychology and the Intellectual Disabilities Faculty of the Royal College of Psychiatrists (2015) 'Dementia and People with Intellectual Disabilities: Guidance on the assessment, diagnosis, interventions and support of people with intellectual disabilities who develop dementia.' Accessed on 4 October 2017 at www.bps.org.uk/system/files/Public%20files/rep77_dementia_and_id.pdf

11

Law, ethics and safeguarding in dementia care

Good health and social care for the vulnerable is a moral imperative, while cost-effective care is an economic one.

How duty of care contributes to safe practice

In tort law, a duty of care is a legal obligation which is imposed on an individual, requiring adherence to a standard of reasonable care while performing any acts that could foreseeably harm others. The landmark case for the UK is *Donoghue v Stevenson* (1932),[1] which established the modern concept of negligence arising from a breach of duty of care, by setting out general principles whereby one person would owe a duty of care to another person.

You have a duty of care to all those receiving care and support in your workplace. This means promoting wellbeing and making sure that people are kept safe from harm, abuse and injury.

Wellbeing could be defined as the positive ways in which a person feels and thinks about themselves. The regulatory code of conduct, according to profession, tells you how you are expected to behave.

Your duty of care is also to other workers – for example, in a hospital, to doctors, nurses and healthcare support workers but also to caterers, cleaners and maintenance workers. If you are a home care worker, you will probably work alone in a variety of homes, but there may well be other people in the premises, as well as the person you are there to support.

Your duty of care is to each individual and to the other workers you come into contact with in the community.

It is important that you have the knowledge and skills to act on your duty of care in your role but that you don't work beyond it. As part of your duty of care, you should pass on any concerns you have about wellbeing.

The agreed ways of working vary from one workplace to another, so you need to check them if you move to a new job in social care or health. Agreed ways of working should be documented, but even if you are told about them only in conversation, you must still work to them.

Dilemmas that may arise between the duty of care and an individual's rights and care partner's wishes

When professionals suspect that a person with dementia is suffering harm from a care partner or other family member or friend, they have both a legal and an ethical duty to act to protect the person with dementia as a 'vulnerable adult'.

Although a careful assessment may sometimes lead to the conclusion that the only way to protect the person's interests is by removing them from their current home, this outcome should never be *assumed* in advance.

The autonomy and wellbeing interests of the person with dementia may be highly complex, and any benefits associated with a long-standing relationship must be weighed in the balance along with the nature and extent of the harm.

Effective communication about proposed treatment or care to enable people with dementia to make informed choices as far as practicable

To promote the dignity of all individuals, they should be fully involved in any decision that affects their care, including personal decisions (such as what to eat, what to wear and what time to go to bed) and wider decisions about their care or support.

Choices can only be made if people have information. If they know the options, the risks and possible implications, they can make the choice that is right for them. This is 'informed' choice.

Sometimes decisions are difficult even when an individual has all the information available.

There are a number of ways that you could help the individual to make informed choices. You can explain information, find people who can share their experiences or ask for the help of specialist workers.

Sometimes an individual may not be able to understand and retain the information they need to make a decision or communicate their choice. If this is the case, they may lack the mental capacity to make the decision. The individual may be able to make day-to-day decisions – for example, what to wear and what they want to eat – but not able to make complex decisions. In situations where you are not entirely sure about the individual's capacity, you should seek additional advice or guidance.

Where possible, people must be supported to make their own decisions. The kinds of support people with dementia may need include:

- making sure their hearing aid is working or they have their glasses on

- explaining things in a way that is easy to understand

- having someone who can speak the person's own language to explain the decision to them

- choosing the best time of the day to talk about the decision.

A person's capacity to consent may be affected by factors such as emotional upset, fatigue, pain or medication. However, the existence of such factors should not lead one to assume that the person lacks the capacity to consent.

All practical and appropriate steps must be made to give a patient the best chance of being able to make a decision for themselves.

The following should be considered:

- Ensure all relevant information has been provided.

- Ensure that this information has been presented in a way that makes it as easy as reasonably possible for the patient to understand.

- Can the patient environment be altered to one more conducive to making a valid consent decision?

Protocols regarding consent to treatment or care for people who may lack mental capacity

People may have capacity to consent to some interventions but not to others, or may have capacity at some times but not others.

Under the Mental Capacity Act 2005, a person must be assumed to have capacity unless it is established that they lack capacity. If there is any doubt, the healthcare professional should assess the capacity of the patient to take the decision in question. This assessment and the conclusions drawn from it should be recorded in the patient's notes.

The Mental Capacity Act also requires that all practical and appropriate steps are taken to enable a person to make the decision themselves. These steps include the following:

- providing relevant information

- communicating in an appropriate way

- making the person feel at ease

- supporting the person.[2]

Independent Mental Capacity Advocates

The Mental Capacity Act provides that an Independent Mental Capacity Advocate (IMCA) must be instructed to represent a person who lacks the requisite capacity, when it is proposed that the person should receive 'serious medical treatment' or be provided with long-term accommodation in a hospital or care home by the NHS or residential care by a local authority.

The duty to instruct an IMCA applies if there is no person (other than a professional or paid care partner) who can be consulted in determining the person's best interests.

IMCAs have prescribed statutory functions, including gathering evidence and preparing a report on the person's best interests.

A person who is subject to a Deprivation of Liberty Safeguards (DoLS) authorisation will also have rights to an IMCA in certain circumstances.

How 'best interests' decisions may need to be made for those lacking capacity

Where it has been decided that a person with dementia is unable to make a decision for themselves, care staff must do what is in the person's best interests. This is known as a best interests decision.

When deciding what is in the person's best interests, you need to:

- involve the person in the decision as much as possible: find out what their views and wishes are (including those they had before they lost capacity to make the decision) and, where possible, involve the person in all meetings where decisions are being made about them

- respect their culture, including their religious beliefs

- talk to people who know them well: this could include family and friends, but also those care staff who have a good knowledge of the person

- try to limit restrictions on the person.

While care staff will not make decisions about what treatment a person with dementia has, they are often involved in giving the treatment – for example, supporting the person to take medication or to apply cream.

When this happens, care staff must have a reasonable belief that either:

- the person has asked for help with their treatment or

- the person lacks capacity to make a decision about the treatment and it is being given in their best interests.

If a doctor has prescribed the treatment to a person with dementia, this would be enough of a basis for care staff to have a reasonable belief that the treatment is in the person's best interests.

If a person often resists the treatment to the extent that they need restraining, the manager of the care home or support service should ask the doctor to reconsider the best interests decision and look for any potential less restrictive options.

How advance decisions can be used to provide information about the wishes of an individual

An advance decision (sometimes known as an advance decision to refuse treatment, an ADRT, or a living will) is a decision you can make now to refuse a specific type of treatment at some time in the future.

An advance decision is *only* legally binding as long as it complies with the Mental Capacity Act and meets a number of specific conditions.

It lets family, care partners and health professionals know whether a person wants to refuse specific treatments in the future. This means they will know an IWD's wishes if he or she is unable to make or communicate those decisions himself or herself.

As long as it is valid and applies to the person's situation, an advance decision gives the health and social care team clinical and legal instructions about a person's treatment choices.

The treatments a person is deciding to refuse must all be named in the advance decision.

A person may want to refuse a treatment in some situations, but not others. If this is the case, the person needs to be clear about all the circumstances in which he or she wants to refuse this treatment.

A person can refuse a treatment that could potentially keep you him or her alive (known as 'life-sustaining treatment').

Deciding to refuse a treatment is not the same as asking someone to end your life or to help you end your life. Euthanasia and assisted suicide are illegal under English law.

Life-sustaining treatment is treatment that replaces or supports ailing bodily functions. For example, a mechanical ventilator can help you to breathe, or taking antibiotics can help your body fight infection.

The range of factors which may indicate neglect, abusive or exploitative practice

Abuse of elders takes many different forms, some involving intimidation or threats against the elderly, some involving neglect, and others involving financial trickery. The most common are defined below.

- **Physical elder abuse**: non-accidental use of force against an elderly person that results in physical pain, injury, or impairment.

- **Emotional elder abuse**: speaking to or treating elderly persons in ways that cause emotional pain or distress.

- **Sexual elder abuse**: contact with an elderly person without the elder's consent.

- **Elder neglect or abandonment by care partners.**

- **Financial exploitation**: unauthorised use of an elderly person's funds or property. An unscrupulous care partner might, for example:

  - misuse an elder's personal cheques, credit cards or accounts

  - steal cash, income cheques or household goods

  - engage in identity theft.

What to do if neglect, abusive or exploitative practice is suspected, including how to raise concerns within local safeguarding or whistleblowing procedures

BOX 11.1 NATIONAL OCCUPATIONAL STANDARDS ON SAFEGUARDING

National Occupational Standard H5SO 04 (SCDHSC0035) – 'Promote the Safeguarding of Individuals' – identifies the requirements associated with safeguarding that must permeate all your work with individuals.

National Occupational Standard SCDLMCB1 – 'Lead and manage practice that promotes the safeguarding of individuals' – identifies the requirements associated with safeguarding which must permeate all your work with individuals and in managing others.

Whistleblowing is the reporting of unsafe or illegal practices in the workplace. Most organisations have a policy or agreed ways of working which will tell you how to raise your concerns. Your employer should provide or explain their whistleblowing policy. You have a responsibility to report things that you feel are not right or are illegal, or if anyone at work is neglecting their duties. Speaking to you manager will normally be your first step.

BOX 11.2 HEALTH AND SOCIAL CARE ACT 2008 (REGULATED ACTIVITIES) REGULATIONS 2014

Regulation 13: The intention of this regulation is to safeguard people who use services from suffering any form of abuse or improper treatment while receiving care and treatment. Improper treatment includes discrimination or unlawful restraint, which includes inappropriate deprivation of liberty under the terms of the Mental Capacity Act 2005.

To meet the requirements of this regulation, providers must have a zero-tolerance approach to abuse, unlawful discrimination and restraint. This includes:

- neglect
- subjecting people to degrading treatment
- unnecessary or disproportionate restraint
- deprivation of liberty.

Providers must have robust procedures and processes to prevent people using the service from being abused by staff or other people they may have contact with when using the service, including visitors.

Abuse and improper treatment includes care or treatment that is degrading for people and care or treatment that significantly disregards their needs or that involves inappropriate recourse to restraint.

For these purposes, restraint includes the use or threat of force and physical, chemical or mechanical methods of restricting liberty to overcome a person's resistance to the treatment in question.

Where any form of abuse is suspected, occurs, is discovered or is reported by a third party, the provider must take appropriate action without delay. The action they must take includes investigation and/or referral to the appropriate body. This applies whether the third party reporting an occurrence is internal or external to the provider.

The Care Quality Commission (CQC) can prosecute for a breach of some parts of this regulation (13(1) to 13(4)) if a failure to meet those parts results in avoidable harm to a person using the service or if a person using the service is exposed to significant risk of harm.

The CQC must refuse registration if providers cannot satisfy them that they can and will continue to comply with this regulation.

The Care Act 2014 sets out a clear legal framework for how local authorities and other parts of the system should protect adults at risk of abuse or neglect.

Local authorities have new safeguarding duties. They must, for example, lead a multiagency local adult safeguarding system that seeks to prevent abuse and neglect, and stop it quickly when it happens; or make enquiries, or request others to make them, when they think an adult with care and support needs may be at risk of abuse or neglect and they need to find out what action may be needed.

The options available when informed consent may be compromised

Obtaining the patient's consent is usually a prerequisite of any clinical intervention.

However, some cognitively impaired patients may not be able to give valid consent. Following years of consultation and legislative review, the Mental Capacity Act 2005 (MCA) provides a statutory framework of 'best interests' decision-making on behalf of incapacitated individuals.

Prevailing confusion and risk-averse practices might mean that the rights and interests of cognitively impaired individuals continue to be compromised, with evidence to suggest that 'best interests' may be conflated with the clinician's evaluation of 'best medical interests'.

This principle is upheld in law and means that medical interventions will generally be unlawful in the absence of the patient's consent, regardless of how unwise or unjustified the patient's decision may appear.

Responding to safeguarding alerts/referrals

Once a safeguarding concern/alert/referral has been raised, it is the host authority's responsibility to lead the initial response in consultation with the funding/placing authority. However, in some circumstances it may be necessary for the host authority to take immediate action to protect the adult at risk (e.g. contact the police or other emergency services).

If – as part of the initial protection plan – the adult is moved to a place of safety, funding responsibilities remain with the funding/placing authority.

This initial protection plan will be reviewed throughout the investigation process.

In consultation with the funding/placing authority, the host authority will seek, where appropriate, medical assessment of any injuries/concerns.

The host authority will coordinate the safeguarding process. This will include gathering information regarding the incident, undertaking background checks of the provider and/or individuals involved, and promptly notifying the funding/placing authority and other relevant agencies.

The funding/placing authority has responsibility to make sure that liaison takes place with the adult at risk/family/care partner/advocate as agreed during the safeguarding adults process.

This might include, for example, informing and updating them regarding the safeguarding adults process, informing and updating them regarding the progress of the investigation, or perhaps identifying a safeguarding liaison person who will take responsibility for ensuring actions are fed back to the host authority during the investigation process.[3]

Evidence-based approaches and techniques to assess neglect or abuse

In the last few years, the issue of abuse and neglect against older people has gained importance at European and national levels.

The World Health Organization and the International Network of the Prevention of Elder Abuse have recognised the abuse of older people as a significant global problem.[4]

Elder abuse has been associated with a number of negative consequences such as reduced quality of life, negative health outcomes, suicidality and a greater mortality.

Prevention of elder maltreatment is a common challenge across governments and many sectors. Public authorities, policy makers, care providers and end users' organisations are more and more aware that, just like child abuse, elder abuse can no longer be tolerated. Measures must be put in place to ensure that all older persons who become dependent on others for care and assistance are adequately protected and can enjoy a dignified old age.

Older people in need of care and assistance, in particular those with complex dependency needs, are considered to be extremely vulnerable to elder abuse and violation of their fundamental rights.

Although a number of instruments have been detected, more research is needed to learn how to better fine-tune assessments and screening tools, to improve initial diagnosing and accuracy in findings.

Such an instrument developed will provide the possibility of early detection of elder abuse which is needed in order to provide support and care, and to prevent more serious levels or an aggravation of elder abuse.

The roles and responsibilities of the different agencies involved in investigating allegations of neglect or abuse

BOX 11.3 DIFFERENT AGENCIES AND SAFEGUARDING

Local authorities

The welfare and protection of vulnerable adults is the corporate responsibility of each and every local authority working in partnership with other public agencies, the voluntary sector and service users and contracted services.

Social services

Social work employers are responsible for identifying situations where a registered, experienced social worker should become involved. Intervention may occur on either a preventive or statutory basis when vulnerable adults and children need safeguarding from abuse, neglect or exploitation, and possibly need removing from their home.

The Care Act 2014 sets out a clear legal framework for how local authorities and other parts of the system should protect adults at risk of abuse or neglect.

Health providers

In planning for most hospital and family health services, there must be assurances that the services provided through commissioning have the appropriate procedures and policies in place to protect the vulnerable adult in all care settings from health providers.

Independent and voluntary sector

Independent and voluntary sector organisations have a responsibility to report any suspicions of abuse to the appropriate agencies, as determined by these procedures.

Police service

The police service has a primary duty and responsibility to protect life and property, to prevent crime and to uphold the law of the land.

National Probation Service

The National Probation Service has a statutory duty to supervise offenders effectively in order to reduce offending and protect the public.

Crown Prosecution Service

The Crown Prosecution Service (CPS) was set up in 1986 by the Prosecution of Offences Act 1985. In accordance with the Act, the CPS is responsible for the prosecution of all criminal cases resulting from police investigations in England and Wales, with the exception of certain minor offences.

Housing support organisations

Housing support organisations that offer tenancy and other support services will include local authorities as landlords, housing associations, voluntary housing organisations and organisations that are managing agents as distinct from landlords.

Victim support organisations

Clients can be referred to victim support if they are in need of support and practical assistance which includes advocacy and liaison around their experiences of any crime.

The importance of sharing safeguarding information with the relevant agencies

Adults have a general right to independence, choice and self-determination, including control over information about themselves. In the context of adult safeguarding, these rights can be overridden in certain circumstances.

Emergency or life-threatening situations may warrant the sharing of relevant information with the relevant emergency services without consent.

The law does not prevent the sharing of sensitive, personal information between organisations where the public interest served outweighs the public interest served by protecting confidentiality – for example, where a serious crime may be prevented.

The Data Protection Act 1998 enables the lawful sharing of information.

There should be a local agreement or protocol in place setting out the processes and principles for sharing information between organisations.

An individual employee cannot give a personal assurance of confidentiality.

Frontline staff and volunteers should always report safeguarding concerns in line with their organisation's policy – this is usually to their line manager in the first instance, except in emergency situations.

It is good practice to try to gain the person's consent to share information. As long as it does not increase risk, practitioners should inform the person if they need to share their information without consent.

The management interests of an organisation should not override the need to share information to safeguard adults at risk of abuse.

Defining 'capacity'

The Mental Capacity Act (MCA) is based on five key principles:

- Every adult has the right to make decisions for themselves. It must be assumed that they are able to make their own decisions unless it has been shown otherwise.

- Every adult has the right to be supported to make their own decisions. All reasonable help and support should be given to assist a person to make their own decisions and communicate those decisions, before it can be assumed that they have lost capacity.

- Every adult has the right to make decisions that may appear to be unwise or strange to others.

- If a person lacks capacity, any decisions taken on their behalf must be in their best interests.

- If a person lacks capacity, any decisions taken on their behalf must be the option least restrictive to their rights and freedoms.

Barriers to sharing concerns

The barriers to care partners sharing concerns are likely to be similar to those identified in relation to other comments and concerns mechanisms within health and social care.

A very good document published by the Association of Directors of Adult Social Services (ADASS) describes how these barriers may shape care partner responses to safeguarding concerns.[5]

Issues relating to understanding and awareness

- Lack of awareness or being unsure if it is wrong or not; being unclear about rights and standards or what 'abuse' means.

- Organisational and staff attitudes to concerns – defensive not responsive.

Issues relating to communication

- Uncertainty about who to go to, how to do so and opportunities to do so.

- Lack of someone to talk to or a source of trusted advice and support.

- Language and literacy barriers.

Deprivation of liberty safeguards

Examples of making decisions or placing restriction on someone with dementia could include deciding on the person's routine, stopping them from walking about at night or preventing them from leaving.

Care home or hospital staff should make sure that all care a person receives involves as little restriction as possible. However, sometimes it will be necessary to take away some of the person's freedom to provide them with the care they need.

Sometimes, taking away a person's freedom in this way can amount to a 'deprivation of liberty'.

A useful definition is that a deprivation of liberty occurs when: 'The person is under continuous supervision and control and is not free to leave, and the person lacks capacity to consent to these arrangements.'[6]

Professionals must follow strict processes called the Deprivation of Liberty Safeguards (DoLS). DoLS are a set of checks that are designed to ensure that a person who is deprived of their liberty is protected, and that this course of action is both appropriate and in the person's best interests.

The definition of what counts as a deprivation of liberty is wide, and so most people with dementia living in care homes and hospitals will receive care that falls under the definition. DoLS offer protection to ensure that when someone's freedom is restricted, it is both in their best interests and, where possible, done in the least restrictive way.

The key elements of these safeguards are:

- to provide the person with a representative – a person who is given certain rights and who should look out for and monitor the person receiving care

- to give the person (or their representative) the right to challenge a deprivation of liberty through the Court of Protection

- to provide a mechanism for a deprivation of liberty to be reviewed and monitored regularly.

The European Court of Human Rights (ECtHR) has confirmed that a deprivation of liberty for the purposes of Article 5(1) of the European Convention on Human Rights has three elements, which apply in all cases:

1. the objective element of confinement in a restricted space for a non-negligible period of time

2. the subjective element that the person has not validly consented to that confinement and

3. the detention being imputable to the state.

In most of the key cases before the ECtHR, it has been common ground that consent is absent and that the state has responsibility; therefore, most attention has been focused on the objective element. ECtHR case law operates on the *Guzzardi* principle that the starting point in assessing whether there has been a deprivation of liberty is 'the concrete situation' of the person and the consideration of 'a whole range of criteria such as the type, duration, effects and manner of implementation of the [restrictive] measure in question'.[7]

Approaches to decision-making

There are some broad approaches to decision-making:

- Valid choice

    - contemporaneous valid choice

    - prior (advance) valid and applicable choice.

- Hypothetical choice (substituted judgement).

- Best interests.

Best interests

The best interests principle of the MCA promotes a holistic view of a person's life, and lays out a process to help a 'lead' decision-maker to make a decision, taking into account what the individual who lacks capacity would have wanted if they had been able to make their own decision.

Why does the MCA not define the underlying concept (or objective) of best interests in terms of the advance decision the person might have made?

There are arguably three possible reasons for rejecting this approach:

1. The first, which could be consistent with the approach of the MCA, is to argue that it is not helpful to try to judge what the person might have written in an advance decision.

2. A second reason is to argue that in understanding this definition the notions of 'valid' and 'applicable' are so crucial that it is not helpful to base the definition (or objective) of best interests on a putative advance decision without a much more detailed understanding of these notions.

3. The third reason for rejecting a conception of best interests based on the external sense of substituted judgement is a rejection of the principle that a valid and applicable advance decision must always be determinative.

Complex situations can also arise in which the best interests of family members or care partners have to be considered alongside those of the person lacking capacity.

Surrogate decision-making

As dementia progresses, many people will reach a stage where they are no longer able to make decisions for themselves.

At this point, decisions about lifestyle, healthcare, medical treatments and end-of-life care become the responsibility of someone else – referred to as a substitute, proxy or surrogate decision-maker (SDM).

There are many ethical issues for family members and others, not least of which is how to negotiate the complexities of decision-making in a way that supports the person's right to make autonomous choices and promotes their quality of life.

Legislation that gives guidance on who would be an appropriate SDM varies from country to country, and sometimes even within a country.

In the UK, a lasting power of attorney – regarding health and welfare and/or property and financial affairs – allows adults with mental capacity to appoint one or more people to help make decisions or make decisions on the person's behalf.

In cases where no legal representative has been appointed, a family member usually assumes the role of informal SDM.

Legal powers

Legal powers are needed before making best interest decisions about the money or property of a person with dementia. There are three possibilities.

Lasting power of attorney

Adults can give someone else the power to make decisions about their money and property. This is called making a lasting power of attorney (property and affairs).

Lasting powers of attorney (LPAs) let you choose a person (or people) you trust to act for you. This person is referred to as your 'attorney', and you can choose what decisions they are allowed to make for you.

There are two different types of LPA. One covers decisions about property and finances, and the other covers decisions about health and welfare. You can choose to make both types or just one. You can appoint the same person to be your attorney for both, or you can have different attorneys.

Deputy

If someone has lost capacity to make some financial decisions, an application can be made to the Court of Protection to appoint someone to look after his or her money. This person is called a 'property and affairs deputy'. Usually, this will be a relative or solicitor. They must act in the person's best interests. (Also, a 'personal welfare deputy' can make decisions about medical treatment and how someone is looked after.)

Appointee

The Department for Work and Pensions can appoint someone else to receive a person's benefits and to use that money to pay for expenses such as household bills, food, personal items and residential accommodation charges. Appointees can only make decisions about the money received in benefits.

UN Convention on the Rights of Persons with Disabilities

The UN Convention on the Rights of Persons with Disabilities (UNCRPD) was ratified by the United Kingdom in 2009. The UNCRPD's purpose is to protect the rights of people who have long-term physical, mental, intellectual or sensory impairments. Although not directly incorporated into UK domestic law, it is applied both by the European Court of Human Rights and domestic courts as an aid to interpretation of the European Convention of Human Rights.

The UNCRPD has been lauded as a new paradigm and as a revolution in human rights law for persons with disabilities.

Its stated purpose is 'to promote, protect and ensure the full and equal enjoyment of all human rights and fundamental freedoms by all persons with disabilities, and to promote respect for their inherent dignity'.[8]

The UNCRPD has a wide field of application and encompasses civil and political rights as well as economic, social and cultural ones.

These rights are extensive and cover matters such as the right to life, access to justice, independent living, education, work and cultural life. Two Articles of the UNCRPD are particularly relevant for the purposes of mental capacity law and the DoLS.

Article 12 sets out the right of persons with disabilities to enjoy to legal capacity on an equal basis with others.[9]

Article 14 stipulates that the 'existence of a disability shall in no case justify a deprivation of liberty'.[10]

The main impetus for supported decision-making schemes has been the UNCRPD.

In particular, Article 12 (the right of disabled people to enjoy legal capacity on an equal basis with others) has been interpreted by the UN Committee on the Rights of Persons with Disabilities as indicating that national laws should provide support to people with disabilities to ensure that their will and preferences are respected, rather than overruled by action that is considered to be in the person's objective best interests.

DoLS are unlikely to comply with Article 14 of the UNCRPD as interpreted by the UN Committee, which contends that any deprivation of liberty on the basis of a person's actual or perceived impairment (even where there are other reasons, including their risk to themselves) amounts to unlawful deprivation of liberty.

The *Bournewood* judgement[11] concerned a man with learning difficulties, who lacked capacity to consent to admission to hospital but who was admitted in his best interests and did not object to being there. The court determined that informal delineation of best interests by health and social care professionals, without right to review or appeal, was in breach of his human rights.

Notes

1. See www.scottishlawreports.org.uk/resources/dvs/donoghue-v-stevenson-report.html
2. Department of Health (2009) 'Reference guide to consent for examination or treatment (second edition).' Accessed on 4 October 2017 at www.gov.uk/government/publications/reference-guide-to-consent-for-examination-or-treatment-second-edition
3. See, for example, Social Care Institute for Excellence (2012) 'Protecting adults at risk: Good practice guide.' Accessed on 4 October 2017 at www.scie.org.uk/publications/adultsafeguardinglondon/files/sections/cross-borough-protocol.pdf
4. World Health Organization, 'Elder abuse.' Accessed on 4 October 2017 at www.who.int/ageing/projects/elder_abuse/en
5. ADASS (2011) 'Carers and safeguarding adults – working together to improve outcomes.' Accessed on 4 October 2017 at http://static.carers.org/files/carers-and-safeguarding-document-june-2011-5730.pdf
6. Alzheimer's Society, 'Deprivation of Liberty Safeguards (DoLS).' Accessed on 4 October 2017 at www.alzheimers.org.uk/info/20032/legal_and_financial/129/deprivation_of_liberty_safeguards_dols/2
7. Guzzardi v Italy (7367/76) [1980] ECHR 5. Accessed on 7 November 2017 at https://publications.parliament.uk/pa/ld200607/ldjudgmt/jd071031/homejj-2.htm
8. UNCRPD, Article 1 – Purpose. Accessed on 4 October 2017 at www.un.org/development/desa/disabilities/convention-on-the-rights-of-persons-with-disabilities/article-1-purpose.html
9. UNCRPD, Article 12 – Equal recognition before the law. See www.un.org/development/desa/disabilities/convention-on-the-rights-of-persons-with-disabilities/article-12-equal-recognition-before-the-law.html

10. UNCRPD, Article 14 – Liberty and security of person. Accessed on 4 October 2017 at www. un.org/development/desa/disabilities/convention-on-the-rights-of-persons-with-disabilities/ article-14-liberty-and-security-of-person.html

11. *HL v United Kingdom* (45508/99) [2004] ECHR 471. There is a useful case summary on the 1COR website, accessed on 4 October 2017 at www.1cor.com/1315/?form_1155. replyids=952

12

End-of-life dementia care

The use of end-of-life care pathways and individualised care plans taking into account psychosocial needs

The starting point is, unfortunately, the huge reluctance to view dementia as a terminal condition.[1] There is no simple way to define the start of the end-of-life care pathway. Some people may be receiving palliative care.

The World Health Organization definition of palliative care describes it as an approach that improves the quality of life of patients and their families facing the problems associated with life-threatening illness.

This is done through the prevention and relief of suffering by means of early identification and impeccable assessment and treatment of pain and other problems, physical, psychosocial and spiritual.

A person living with long-term conditions will be under continual review for deterioration of their condition.

Making decisions about end-of-life care and treatment on behalf of a family member may be difficult.

Goals of care in palliative and end-of-life care pathways will need to be changed when appropriate. Palliative care gives less priority to survival and independence, and it acknowledges the fragility and interdependence of individual existence and that vulnerability is shared with caregivers. Families may be apprehensive about making decisions about future care and will want to seek the best course of action for their relative in an uncertain situation.

Family care partners' patterns of decision-making differ according to their previous experiences of end-of-life care, education, perceived care partner stress, psychological distress and cultural background. Not surprisingly, care partners often find making health-related decisions for the person they care for stressful. Decisions concerning end-of-life care are among the most difficult.

Families who are in conflict or with poor inter-relational dynamics may be more likely to opt for active treatment rather than palliative care.

However, even in the absence of such conflict, when a family is in doubt or uncertain as to what to decide, they may err on the side of caution and elect for life-sustaining treatment for the person with dementia.

Advance care planning (ACP)

An issue that could prompt ACP discussions is a decline in mental capacity, such as through dementia or delirium. The Mental Capacity Act 2005 (MCA) governs decision-making on behalf of adults who lack the capacity to make some or all decisions for themselves. The Act came into force in 2007.

The capacity of individuals to talk through and express their wishes diminishes as dementia advances, and ACP is not considered routinely as part of dementia services early in the disease pathway. The National Dementia Strategy and a report commissioned by the Alzheimer's Society advocate timely ACP.

ACP has been defined as a process of discussion between an individual, their care providers and often those close to them, about future care.

The difference between ACP and general planning is that the purpose of ACP is to make clear the person's preferences and wishes in the context of their condition deteriorating and the likely loss of their capacity to make decisions or communicate their wishes to others. It is advised that the results of ACP discussions are documented and regularly reviewed, and, with the person's permission, are communicated to everyone who may be involved their care.

The discussion may lead to:

- an advance statement (a statement of wishes and preferences)

- an advance decision to refuse treatment (ADRT – a specific refusal of treatment(s) in a predefined potential future situation)

- the appointment of a personal welfare lasting power of attorney (LPA).

Advance decisions and statements

An advance decision[2] to refuse treatment lets you, while you have mental capacity, make a decision about medical treatment(s) you would want to refuse, should you at some time in the future lack mental capacity to decide and/or express your wishes when the decision needs to be made.

An advance statement allows you to make more general statements, describing your wishes and preferences about future care should you be unable to make or communicate a decision or express your preferences at the time. You may want it to reflect your religious or other beliefs and important aspects of your life.

How to recognise and manage pain in people with advanced dementia

Pain is one of the most common symptoms that people with dementia experience. However, often it is poorly recognised and undertreated in dementia.

A main reason for this is that, as dementia progresses, the person's ability to communicate their needs becomes more difficult.

Attention to non-verbal communication is vital to understand the world of individuals who can no longer put their feelings across in words reliably; relationships cannot develop without communication, and quality care is impossible without relationships.

Research on the assessment of pain for people with end-stage dementia is limited and has focused on the ability of care partners to predict pain and the validity and perceived usefulness of different pain assessment tools for end-of-life care.

The widely accepted definition of pain was developed by a taxonomy task force of the International Association for the Study of Pain: 'Pain is an unpleasant sensory and emotional experience that is associated with actual or potential tissue damage or described in such terms.'

Pain is a very personal thing. This means that – as the International Association of Hospice and Palliative Care says – 'pain is what the person says hurts'[3]: that is, it is what the person describes and feels as pain. No other person can experience the pain, know what it feels like or how it really affects the person physically and emotionally.

There are a number of reasons why people with dementia typically receive poor pain relief.

- The most obvious is that the person with dementia may lose the ability to communicate that they are in pain.

- Also, care partners and care staff often do not recognise when a person is in pain or do not know how to help.

- People may think that some behaviours – for example, calling out for help repeatedly – are due to 'the dementia' rather than to pain.

- Some believe that people with dementia do not experience pain or that because their memory is so poor they forget the experience.

Many older people live with dementia, and therefore many of the causes of pain will be the same for all older people. It is important to be very clear on whether the person has any other conditions – for example, osteoarthritis, ulcers, pressure sores, recent injuries or fractures.

People often experience pain when a part of the body is moving, so, for example, a person is most likely to experience pain when they are being helped to turn in bed, get dressed or undressed, or when a wound dressing is being changed.

How can we know if the person is in pain? The best thing to do is to ask the person directly. Many people with moderate or even advanced dementia may still be able to provide information on their pain. Keep questions simple, as some people may not understand what you mean when you use the word 'pain'. You may need to ask questions such as 'Is it sore?' or 'Does it hurt?'

When a person has poor short-term memory, they may only be able to tell you if they are in pain at that moment – they may not remember if they had pain five minutes or five hours ago.

Asking how severe pain is may also be difficult: 'Does it hurt a lot?' or 'How much?' may not be helpful, as often the person will not be able to describe how bad the pain is or how often it occurs.

Use a tested tool to assess pain

A number of different resources are available to help care staff establish whether a person with dementia is in pain, especially if the person cannot tell you in words.[4]

Assessment of pain, by observing behaviour in those who are unable to communicate verbally, can identify the presence of distress, but cannot differentiate it from other forms of anguish. Pain assessment tools are available to help identify pain when individuals can no longer reliably communicate this verbally.

A 'tested tool' can guide you to the cause of the pain, its severity, when it occurs and what helps to make the pain better or worse. It will give you evidence to show a nurse or doctor if the pain is present or gone. If the pain is still present, always inform a doctor or nurse to review the person's medication.

Even where pain is suspected and reported by formal or informal care partners, communication of this to medical staff is not always effective in achieving prescription of analgesia. Lack of consideration of the possibility of pain as a cause of behaviour changes may be responsible for this.

Some people with advanced dementia, who may no longer understand the connection between taking analgesia and relief of pain, may be unwilling to accept oral medication. This can occur even when signs of pain are clearly present and can lead to care partner stress and patient distress during frequent confrontations regarding taking medication.

One of the most common and effective medicines to relieve pain in advanced dementia is paracetamol. Paracetamol can be given one hour before someone is helped to move or before a dressing needs to be changed. If paracetamol fails, then stronger drugs can be tried, although these may have side effects (including increased confusion) and should be carefully monitored.

Other medications to relieve pain include antibiotics to treat infection, laxatives to relieve constipation, antacids or alginates to help indigestion, and peppermint water to relieve wind-type pain.

You can ask a range of professionals for advice on pain management: a tissue viability nurse, palliative care or district nurse, physiotherapist or massage therapist, or a GP or pain specialist team in your local area.

Other ways to tackle pain, without medication, include gentle exercises and careful positioning in a bed or chair.

Identification of symptoms associated with end of life and how these symptoms can be managed with care and compassion

Effective communication becomes more difficult as dementia progresses, and both expressive and receptive language abilities are affected.

Environmental factors and staff or care partner ability to listen, interpret and communicate effectively play an important part in quality care.

Pain

Some people assume that people with dementia don't feel pain, but this is not true. If a person with dementia is in pain, and this is not recognised and treated properly, they may become very distressed.

The following things may help when assessing whether the person is in pain:

- **Knowledge of the person** – there may be certain things that they typically do when they are in pain, such as cry out or become very withdrawn.

- **Observation** – signs that someone is in pain include their behaviour (e.g. being agitated, irritable, tearful or unable to sleep), facial expressions (e.g. grimacing), body language (if they are tense or rocking, or pulling at a particular part of their body) and vocalisations (e.g. shouting out, screaming and moaning).

- **Bodily changes** – a high temperature, sweating or looking very pale can also indicate pain.

Eating and drinking

Issues of nutrition become complex and ethically challenging in relation to a person with dementia as the end of life approaches.

Swallowing problems are a common reason for reduced food intake and malnutrition.

These leave the person vulnerable to aspiration pneumonia and may be an indication that the end-of-life phase of dementia is approaching.

Other reasons include reduced appetite and enjoyment of food, increased sleep or agitation, and/or unvoiced and undetected discomfort.

These symptoms cause distress to family and/or care partners. Problems surrounding artificial feeding and fluid replacement need to be explored with families by staff who have a sound knowledge of the issues, enabling informed choices to be made between artificial feeding and comfort feeding only.

Comfort feeding is an approach advocating careful hand feeding, as long as no distress is caused. Someone in the later stages of dementia should be offered food and fluids – even if these are just mouthfuls or sips – for as long as they show an interest and can take them safely.

When a person is close to death, they will usually stop eating and drinking. Relatives might worry that the person is starving or getting dehydrated and not being cared for properly.

People should be prepared to discuss openly matters about food and fluids for the person, including what the person has said or recorded as their wishes. It is important that what is in the person's best interests comes first.

Artificial nutrition and hydration

If a person is struggling to eat and drink enough, and their swallowing is unsafe, artificial nutrition and hydration or 'tube feeding' might be considered. The most widely used treatments are:

- a nasogastric tube which passes down the nose and into the stomach

- a PEG tube which passes directly into the stomach through a hole in the skin.

Each person's situation should be considered individually.

Most healthcare professionals now agree that giving food and fluids artificially is not appropriate if the person's problems with eating, drinking or swallowing are because their dementia is in the later stages.

Infections

People in the later stages of dementia are at greater risk of infections such as urinary tract infections or chest infections (such as pneumonia). These can be caused by lower fluid intake, swallowing problems and reduced mobility.

People disagree about whether antibiotics should be used to treat infections in a person in the later stages of dementia.

It may be appropriate to use antibiotics to ease distress and discomfort at the end of life even if the infection cannot be cured or is likely to happen again.

Think about whether to give antibiotics on an individual basis. In prescribing a drug, consider:

- the likely benefits

- the risk of side effects

- the burden of giving the drugs

- the person's wishes (*if known*).

Feelings

Families go through varying degrees of feelings of loss, depression, anxiety, guilt, frustration and hopelessness, and often they do not get an opportunity to express their feelings as they are too busy caring for the patient and fear being judged.

It is important to provide family care partners with space and time to talk about their own feelings. They should be equipped to deal with anticipatory grief.

Exploring the views and preferences of all stakeholders involved in end-of-life care in dementia is necessary to evaluate current provision and inform how care can be improved.

End of life in young-onset dementia

Young adult care partners of persons with dementia are found to use combinations of strategies including action-oriented, cognitive and emotional strategies that amount to more detachment from their parent with dementia in end-of-life stages.

Studies have demonstrated that children of parents with young onset dementia feel overlooked as individuals and that their needs have been neglected. They are described as travelling a journey 'alone', 'fighting' against health and care services.[5] The children have to be seen and get recognition and support.

The support systems for families of persons with young-onset dementia should be family-oriented, but at the same time individuals who support these families should recognise that all family members have unique personal experiences regarding how dementia has influenced their lives.

The needs of bereaved families and friends including the potential for conflicting emotions

Grief occurs from losses in the quality of the relationship, intimacy, memory, communication, social interaction, health status and opportunities to resolve issues from the past. Ambiguity about the future, anger, frustration and guilt are factors that contribute to care partners' anticipatory grief. This grief is likely to be prolonged due to the progressive nature and extended duration of dementia.

Anticipatory grief is exacerbated by the loss experienced when the person living with dementia is no longer able to remain at home and becomes a resident in a care facility. Finally, family care partners experience grief for the loss upon death of the person with dementia.

It has been well established that caring for a loved one with dementia can be difficult and stressful, potentially leading to a range of negative outcomes for family care partners.

While some family care partners respond with remarkable resilience, others experience varying degrees of depressive symptomatology, anxiety, complicated grief, and other mental health problems. A mixture of conflicting emotions can occur in bereavement and grief.

When a person with dementia experiences a bereavement, they sometimes experience and remember a profound shock and sense of bewilderment. At other times they may not recall or understand the loss, but it can still have a strong emotional impact on them, reflected in their behaviour and mood.

Supporting family and friends to celebrate the life of the deceased person

It can be helpful to celebrate the life of the person with dementia, after he or she has died. It is not uncommon for a local memorial to be arranged, such as some favourite flowers planted in a place of emotional significance. Or else, it can be helpful to give a formal eulogy at a funeral, celebrating aspect of the life of the person with dementia, including his or her time living without dementia.

Good advice is found within an excellent factsheet from Alzheimer's Australia, entitled 'Coping after the death of someone with dementia'.[6] Some points include the following:

- Take time off. The length of time needed to adjust to life changes varies from individual to individual. Be patient and don't try to rush the process.

- Reminiscence can be helpful after a bereavement.

Cultural and religious differences associated with death, care of the dying and the deceased person

Grieving and death rituals vary across cultures and are often heavily influenced by religion.

How and when rituals are practised will vary depending on the country of origin and level of acculturation into the mainstream society.

The duration, frequency and intensity of the grief process may also vary based on the manner of death and the individual family and cultural beliefs.

Although cultural practices surrounding the death of a loved one have been described, there are limited research descriptions from key informants within cultures.

For example, the Hindu view of pain and suffering is very different from Western concepts. Pain and suffering are viewed as part of karma, which is the unfolding of events based on a person's current and previous lives. Put succinctly, pain and suffering are viewed as the state the individual is supposed to be in.

The development of practices and services that meet the end-of-life needs of people with dementia

The training of all staff in hospitals and care homes in the palliative care approach is essential to improve their knowledge and skills in this area. Even if there are ethical and practical difficulties in conducting good-quality research in advanced dementia, there should be no reason not to use a palliative care approach in dementia management.

Palliative care specialists emphasise that identifying and responding to the physical care needs of the individual with dementia must form the cornerstone of any approach.

There are several care models, such as the Gold Standards Framework (GSF), that focus on care in the last year or months of life. GSF is a systematic approach for professionals to provide good-quality care at the end of life, and emphasises good communication, coordination, control of symptoms, continuity, continued learning, care partner support and care of the dying.

There should be regular communication and information-sharing between the family and the professionals involved in care to ensure improved quality of care and avoid confusion, mistrust and mis-understanding so that everyone involved is aware of what is happening.

There is a need to differentiate between the relative effectiveness and suitability of different end-of-life interventions developed for care home populations, and specifically those with dementia.

The processes involved in deciding when a person with dementia is deemed to be at end of life

Recognising when a person stops living with dementia and starts dying from it, and the prediction of survival time, can influence decisions to involve specialist palliative care services and the release of resources.

It can also influence decision-making about the benefit of transferring patients to acute services.

A failure to recognise that someone is dying can result in potentially distressing and unnecessary hospital admissions.

A number of studies indicate that health professionals are not skilled at recognising the end stages of dementia. For example, a US study of 883 nursing home residents found that 1 per cent of people with dementia were recorded as having a life expectancy of less than six months, but 71 per cent of them died during this period.[7]

A Korean study from Suh and colleagues tested the hypothesis that mortality in people with dementia is higher in care homes than in the community and found no difference in mortality rate. Predictors of death were age, global deterioration, duration of disease, the presence of hallucinations, wandering and depression.[8]

Little consensus has so far been found about the value of prognostic indicators for people with dementia. Several studies have tested and validated scales to predict survival.[9]

Dementia-specific advice and guidance on end-of-life care

Improving end-of-life care for people with dementia has been the focus of UK policy and guidance for over a decade now.

However, we still see many examples where people with dementia do not have fair access to palliative and end-of-life care services and support, and where their family care partners do not have access to bereavement support after their death.

A difficulty for services such as hospices is in understanding what it is they can offer to this group of people and when.

Life expectancy is increasing so people often develop a range of conditions and disabilities during the years of old age before death. As dementia is largely a disease of old age, many people with dementia will also have other illnesses or disabilities. Multi-morbidity is characterised by complex interactions of such coexisting diseases where a medical approach focused on a single disease does not suffice.

Multi-morbidity including dementia often presents clinicians with practical problems in following treatment regimes or in understanding prognosis.

Dementia UK, with its Admiral Nursing model,[10] has been developing its own approach for people with dementia and their families to enable those with the disease not only to live well but to die well also. When considering dementia, frailty and complex multi-morbidity, it can be difficult to identify when someone may enter the final stages of their life.

Admiral Nurse Leaders have become very aware that providing good palliative and end-of-life care for people with dementia often combines knowledge, expertise and skills relating to both dementia and palliative and end-of-life care.

Notes

1. For a discussion of this issue, see chapter 12, 'Dying well' in Rahman, S. (2017) *Enhancing Health and Wellbeing in Dementia: A Person-Centred Integrated Care Approach*. London: Jessica Kingsley Publishers, especially pp.296–297.

2. AgeUK, 'Advance decisions, advance statements and living wills.' Factsheet 72, April 2017. Accessed on 4 October at www.ageuk.org.uk/documents/en-gb/factsheets/fs72_advance_decisions_advance_statements_and_living_wills_fcs.pdf?dtrk=true

3. Cited in 'Pain in advanced dementia.' Accessed on 7 November 2017 at https://www.scie.org.uk/dementia/advanced-dementia-and-end-of-life-care/end-of-life-care/pain.asp

4. Examples include the Abbey Pain Scale, NOPPAIN, PACSLAC, PADE, CNPI and PAINAD. These are all reviewed in Lichtner, V., Dowding, D., Esterhuizen, P., Closs, S.J. et al. (2014) 'Pain assessment for people with dementia: a systematic review of systematic reviews of pain assessment tools.' *BMC Geriatr 17*, 14, 138. Accessed on 7 November 2017 at www.ncbi.nlm.nih.gov/pmc/articles/PMC4289543

5. For example, Johannessen, A., Engedal, K. and Thorsen, K. (2015) 'Adult children of parents with young-onset dementia narrate the experiences of their youth through metaphors.' *J Multidiscip Healthc 8*, 245–54.

6. https://act.fightdementia.org.au/support-and-services/families-and-friends/taking-care-of-yourself/coping-after-the-death-of-someone-with-dementia

7. Mitchell, S.L., Kiely, D.K. and Hamel, M.B. (2004) 'Dying with advanced dementia in the nursing home.' *Archives of Internal Medicine 164*, 3, 321–326.

8. Suh, G.H., Kil Yeon, B., Shah, A. and Lee, J.Y. (2005) 'Mortality in Alzheimer's disease: A comparative prospective Korean study in the community and nursing homes.' *International Journal of Geriatric Psychiatry 20*, 1, 26–34.

9. For example, the Advanced Dementia Prognostic Tool (ADEPT): 'A Risk Score to Estimate Survival in Nursing Home Residents with Advanced Dementia.' Accessed on 7 November 2017 at www.ncbi.nlm.nih.gov/pmc/articles/PMC2981683

10. See www.dementiauk.org/get-support/admiral-nursing

13

Research and evidence-based practice in dementia care

This is an exciting time to get involved in research and evidence-based practice in dementia care.

If you look up #whywedoresearch on Twitter, you'll find great examples of research being disseminated. Twitter is an excellent innovation for discussing ideas for research too, as the platform is a combination of mass media and interpersonal communication.

For an excellent discussion of evidence-based healthcare, see Trisha Greenhalgh's *How to Implement Evidence-Based Healthcare.*[1]

The difference between audit, service evaluation and research

There are three main types of projects which can be undertaken:

- research
- service evaluation/survey
- clinical audit.

The main difference between a service evaluation and a clinical audit is that the latter makes reference to a standard whereas the former does not.

Both service evaluation and clinical audit only tend to involve interventions that are well established within the institution, as opposed to a research project which may involve new interventions.

In both service evaluation and clinical audit, the choice of treatment is decided between the clinician and patient, whereas in the case of clinical outcomes-based research a randomisation process is usually used to allocate treatment.

Furthermore, treatment allocation by protocol is only done in the case of a research project. Finally, neither service evaluation nor clinical audits involve a Research Ethics Committee review, whereas a research project typically does.

A summary table explaining the differences is shown below.

Table 13.1 Comparison of research, clinical audit and service provision[2]

Research	Clinical audit	Service evaluation
The attempt to derive generalisable new knowledge including studies that aim to generate hypotheses as well as studies that aim to test them.	Designed and conducted to produce information to inform delivery of best care.	Designed and conducted solely to define or judge current care.
May involve randomisation	No randomisation	No randomisation
Hypothesis-driven	No hypothesis	No hypothesis
Quantitative research is designed to test a hypothesis. Qualitative research identifies/explores themes following established methodology.	Designed to answer the question: 'Does this service reach a predetermined standard?'	Designed to answer the question: 'What standard does this service achieve?'

Participating in service evaluation and research in the workplace

BOX 13.1 NATIONAL OCCUPATIONAL STANDARDS ON RESEARCH

National Occupation Standard R&D8 – 'Conduct investigations in selected research and development topics' – applies to conducting investigations in selected research and development topics. Investigations may be undertaken by a single researcher, a research team, within a single discipline, multidisciplinary or multi-site.

National Occupational Standard R&D11 – 'Record conclusions and recommendations of research and development activities' – covers recording conclusions and recommendations of research and development activities, ensuring that practice reflects up-to-date information and policies.

National Occupational Standard R&D10 – 'Interpret results of research and development activities' – involves the researcher in interpreting results from a single hypothesis, single researcher activity, own research project or as a member of a research team

National Occupational Standard R&D9 – 'Collate and analyse data relating to research' – covers collating and analysing data relating to research, using methods and data types specified in the research proposal. It is expected that the researcher would use methods and data types, which are specified within the research proposal.

National Occupational Standard R&D14 – 'Translate research and development findings into practice' – has broad application. It will involve the conduct of pilot studies and/or field trials following results of research activities.

Researchers who wish to involve those to whom they owe a professional duty of care (such as teachers and their pupils, or doctors and patients) should be especially careful to clarify that there is no perceived pressure to participate, and to ensure that participation cannot have any effect on the professional care provided to the participants (and that the participants are aware of this).

Researchers can use workplace information in their research if they ensure that the role as researcher is separated.

Your workplace is responsible for ensuring compliance with law (e.g. Data Protection Act 1998) and good conduct (e.g. that research with human participants is conducted ethically) for work undertaken within its remit. This includes the provision of anonymous, unidentifiable data to you to use in your capacity as a researcher. You may use anonymous, unidentifiable information provided to you by your workplace if you have permission from your workplace to do this.

One thing evident from different perspectives on involvement and partial history of individual involvement is the range of different motivations that have contributed to it.

These perspectives include the following interrelated approaches:

- a consumerist approach

- a democratic approach

- an ethical and outcomes-based approach

- a value-based approach

- an approach based on sustainability

- a person-centred care approach.

The current state of involvement has arisen from different initiatives led by different groups, at a number of different points in time, influenced by different ideologies and serving different goals. It is not a neat, single concept but encompasses multiple perspectives, which is important to understand when considering how and why people support or resist different forms of involvement.

Policy has tended mainly to focus on or articulate patient involvement in the form of rights, but inherent in this are associated responsibilities.

One of the big difficulties researchers face today is recruiting participants for their studies. At the same time, many people are looking for studies to contribute to and take part in, but don't know where to find out about them. This is why various entities have joined forces to develop Join Dementia Research, a service which allows people to register their interest in participating in dementia research and be matched to suitable studies. Everybody now has that chance to see what dementia research is taking place, both in their local area and across the nation.[3]

How people affected by dementia may be involved in service evaluation and research

In the past, the person with dementia was viewed as a 'disease entity', unable to contribute directly to an understanding of the condition. Such exclusions could frustrate the growth of scientific knowledge, denying future patients and care partners the benefits. Nevertheless, researchers must have a sound justification for including people with dementia: their inclusion must be appropriate for addressing the study's research questions.

The move towards person-centred care has resulted in growing acknowledgement that people with dementia have rights, including the right for their experiences to be explored through research.

Interest in psychological and biographical aspects of the life experiences of people with dementia has been important in this change.

Although a sizable and growing group in our society, it is still common for persons with dementia, in keeping with the wider social and cultural exclusion they experience, to be excluded from service evaluation and qualitative research.

There is an increasing recognition among researchers, particularly within social gerontology and nursing, that persons with dementia should not only be included in research (as subjects) but also be given opportunities to participate in research as subjects. With this comes the accompanying debate around what inclusion in research means and the level to which it can be achieved without being too cognitively and emotionally demanding for persons with dementia.

According to INVOLVE,[4] active public involvement in research would involve people other than researchers:

- helping to identify and ask the right questions in the right way

- ensuring that health and social care research is relevant to patients, service users and the public

- participating in the research process, whether designing, managing, undertaking or disseminating research.

Example of working group involvement: the SDWG

The Scottish Dementia Working Group (SDWG) is a campaigning group of people with dementia. Since 2001, the SDWG has been at the forefront of a growing movement towards people with dementia influencing decisions about their lives.

The SDWG research sub-group, established in August 2013, provides a forum in which the large volume of requests coming into the SDWG to collaborate in research can be considered.

Examples of 'core principles' developed within the ambit of this group are shown in Box 13.2.

BOX 13.2 TWO OUT OF THE SIX CORE PRINCIPLES DEVELOPED BY SDWG[5]

'Researchers should ask people with dementia how they want to be involved in research, including at what points and in what ways they want to be updated. Different people will have different views on this.'

'Researchers should create opportunities for us to develop our research skills so that we can be involved in influencing knowledge about dementia.'

Systematic research methods to facilitate evidence-based practice

Practitioners can save considerable time and rely on someone else's expertise when they are provided with access to pre-filtered evidence. Pre-filtered evidence is established when someone with expertise in a substantive area has reviewed and presented the methodologically strongest data in the field.

Systematic reviews provide practitioners with a vehicle to gain access to such pre-filtered evidence. Essentially, systematic reviews aim to synthesise the results of multiple original studies by using strategies that delimit bias.

According to Petticrew and Roberts, [6] systematic reviews 'adhere closely to a set of scientific methods that explicitly aim to limit systematic error (bias), mainly attempting to identify, appraise and synthesize all relevant studies (of whatever design) in order to answer a particular question (or set of questions)'. Systematic reviews substantially reduce the time and expertise it would take to locate and subsequently appraise and synthesise individual studies.

The range of evidence that informs decision-making, care practice and service delivery

Systematic reviews and meta-analyses have become increasingly important in healthcare. Clinicians read them to keep up to date with their field, and they are often used as a starting point for developing clinical practice guidelines.

Granting agencies may require a systematic review to ensure there is justification for further research, and some healthcare journals are moving in this direction.

A systematic review is a summary of the medical literature that uses explicit and reproducible methods to systematically search, critically appraise and synthesise on a specific issue. It synthesises the results of multiple primary studies related to each other by using strategies that reduce biases and random errors.

To this end, systematic reviews may or may not include a statistical synthesis called meta-analysis depending on whether the studies are similar enough so that combining their results is meaningful.

The evidence-based practitioner David Sackett provides the following definitions:

Review: The general term for all attempts to synthesize the results and conclusions of two or more publications on a given topic.

Overview: When a review strives to comprehensively identify and track down all the literature on a given topic (also called 'systematic literature review').

Meta-analysis: A specific statistical strategy for assembling the results of several studies into a single estimate.[7]

Systematic reviews adhere to a strict scientific design based on explicit, pre-specified and reproducible methods. Because of this, when carried out well, they provide reliable estimates about the effects of interventions so that conclusions are defensible.

Systematic reviews can also demonstrate where knowledge is lacking. This can then be used to guide future research.

Systematic reviews are usually carried out in the areas of clinical tests (diagnostic, screening and prognostic), public health interventions, adverse (harm) effects, economic (cost) evaluations and how and why interventions work.

Cochrane reviews are systematic reviews undertaken by members of the Cochrane Collaboration, which is an international not-for-profit organisation that aims to help people to make well-informed decisions about healthcare by preparing, maintaining and promoting the accessibility of systematic reviews of the effects of healthcare interventions.

A meta-analysis is the combination of data from several independent primary studies that address the same question to produce a single estimate such as the effect of treatment or risk factor. It is the statistical analysis of a large collection of analysis and results from individual studies for the purpose of integrating the findings.

The fundamental rationale of meta-analysis is that it reduces the quantity of data by summarising data from multiple resources and helps to plan research as well as to frame guidelines.

It also helps to make efficient use of existing data, ensuring generalisability, helping to check consistency of relationships, explaining data inconsistency, and quantifies the data. It helps to improve the precision in estimating the risk by using explicit methods.

Approaches to evaluating services and measuring impact, including the use of outcomes reported by people affected by dementia

In any field, improving performance and accountability depends on having a shared goal that unites the interests and activities of all stakeholders.

In healthcare, however, stakeholders have myriad, often conflicting goals, including access to services, profitability, high quality, cost containment, safety, convenience, patient-centredness and satisfaction.

Achieving high value for patients must become the overarching goal of healthcare delivery, with value defined as the health outcomes achieved per dollar spent. This goal is what matters for patients and unites the interests of all actors in the system. If value improves, patients, payers, providers and suppliers can all benefit while the economic sustainability of the overall healthcare system increases.

Since value is defined as outcomes relative to costs, it encompasses efficiency. Cost reduction without regard to the outcomes achieved is dangerous and self-defeating, leading to false 'savings' and potentially limiting effective care.

So far, no standard method – such as bibliometrics – has emerged that can measure the benefit of research to society (i.e. the broader impact of research) reliably and with validity.

Dementia UK's GEANS (Getting Evidence into Admiral Nurse Services) programme collects evidence of how Admiral Nurses contribute to families living with dementia, and how the work of Admiral Nurses promotes best practice in dementia care.[8] The aim of this innovative programme is to expand the published evidence of the effectiveness of Admiral Nursing services and to evaluate critically the added value of their specialist clinical role.

Ethical issues related to conducting research with people who have a cognitive impairment

The need for research into treatment for dementia as well as palliation and care of its symptoms is well recognised.

However, conducting research with people living with dementia brings about a series of ethical concerns surrounding research risks in vulnerable populations which make seeking approval for and conducting studies difficult.

There is further call for protection measures concerning privacy and confidentiality to ensure that research is undertaken with full respect to the human rights of people during the research process. However, the research process can be impeded by a lack of coherent guidance from governing bodies and institutions.

People with cognitive impairments may be routinely excluded from studies due to concerns about safeguarding vulnerabilities and lack of an ability to provide informed consent, which in turn feed into the production of a lack of autonomy for persons with dementia.

Participating in research: informed consent

Before anyone participates in a study, they should have given their informed consent to the researchers or doctors in charge of the study.

Giving informed consent involves more than just acceptance to take part as the decision must be based on a full understanding of what is involved.

The information concerning the study should be provided by the organisers and be understandable to potential participants who should be given time to take in the information and ask any questions. For this reason, informed consent should be seen as a process rather than simply a document to be signed.

Part of the process of informed consent involves finding out what is involved in a specific study and then taking the necessary time to decide when that is acceptable.

For studies involving medical treatment or drugs, the consent procedure is a medico-legal requirement covered by laws and codes of medical ethics.

Consent in case of incapacity or reduced capacity to consent

Many people who are in the early stages of dementia have the capacity to consent to participation in research.

However, it is important that researchers understand that people with dementia may have certain difficulties with comprehension, attention span, memory and communication.

For this reason, researchers need to take extra care to ensure that the information they have given has been understood and to respect each person's pace.

Printed information can be helpful as a support to memory, and going back over what has been said can help the person remember what is involved. Involving a care partner can also be helpful, provided that the person with dementia agrees to this.

Substitute decision-making and research

Sometimes research can only be carried out on people who are in a fairly advanced stage of dementia (e.g. in the case of research into palliative care or for experimental drugs to be used in more advanced stages of dementia). This raises an ethical issue if the person with dementia is no longer able to give fully informed consent.

The provisions of the Convention on Human Rights and Biomedicine (1997) provide for consent to be given on behalf of a person who does not have the capacity to consent. This could be a legal representative or body, or anyone who has the authority to give consent on the person's behalf.[9]

However, the person with dementia should still be involved in the decision-making process as much as possible. In some studies, especially longitudinal ones, a person may have consented at the beginning and lost capacity during the study.

Substitute decision makers (whether healthcare proxies, legal guardians or relatives) could also discuss the issue of research with the person with dementia, speak to the researchers about interpretation of the advance directive, monitor the research process and signal any problems.

It is important that when people designate a healthcare proxy, they discuss their preferences and feelings about different types of care with them, and any views about participation in research.

Principles of disseminating research findings clearly and accurately

There are three interesting National Occupational Standards on presenting research findings.

BOX 13.3 NATIONAL OCCUPATIONAL STANDARDS ON PRESENTING RESEARCH FINDINGS

National Occupational Standard R&D13 – 'Present findings of research and development activities' – applies to the preparation and conduct of oral presentations, which may be presented by the researcher themselves or presented to others in authority as part of a wider presentation of results. It is expected that presentation materials will be fit for purpose and will include bibliography and referencing in line with accepted conventions relevant to the scale and audience for the research findings.

National Occupational Standard R&D15 – 'Evaluate and report on the application of research and development findings within practice' – involves responsibility for evaluating the pilot and field studies and assessing the combined recommendations of research and development projects and associated pilot and field studies. It also involves producing the evaluation report, with recommendations for the relevant target audience.

National Occupational Standard R&D12 – 'Present findings of research and development activities in written form' – applies to the preparation of formal documentation, which may be presented by the researcher themselves or be presented to others in authority as part of a wider presentation of results. It is expected that documentation will include bibliography and referencing in line with accepted conventions relevant to the scale and audience for the research results. The final presented document may range from an internal research report to a more formal document for publication.

A commonly accepted definition of dissemination includes 'to distribute or scatter about'.[10]

> Review past dissemination strategies
> Devise dissemination objectives
> Determine audiences
> Develop messages
> Decide on dissemination approaches
> Determine dissemination channels
> Review available resources
> Consider timing and windows of opportunity
> Evaluate efforts

Figure 13.1 Dissemination efforts[11]

Dissemination tools

Various dissemination tools are available to research teams pursuing the uptake of research findings. All these tools should be considered less as individual pieces and more as parts of a whole. The dissemination tools considered in this module will include, research reports, peer review papers, press releases, and policy briefs.

BOX 13.4 DISSEMINATION TOOLS

Research reports	The content of the research report depends on the grant body and their specific requirements.
Peer review papers	For many researchers, publication in a peer-reviewed journal is a critical outcome.
Press releases	The media is a crucial audience for research findings because it can popularise findings and promote feedback.
Policy briefs	Policy briefs are short documents aimed at a non-specialised audience.

The importance of continuing professional development to ensure the methods used are robust, valid and reliable

A recent definition of continuing professional development (CPD) by the Directors of the CPD Subcommittee of the Academy of Medical Royal Colleges is:

> A continuing process, outside formal undergraduate and postgraduate training, that enables individual doctors to maintain and improve standards of medical practice through the development of knowledge, skills, attitudes and behaviour, CPD should also support specific changes in practice.[12]

The definition of CPD could be divided into two parts:

- gaining knowledge
- improving patient care.

A vital role of CPD is ensuring that everyday practice is best practice. The latter is always informed by research on new knowledge, skills, techniques or innovatory practice.

Learning something new could be described as 'keeping up-to-date' and as 'keeping my practice up-to-date'.

The nature of what is newly learned will vary according to professional roles and from specialty to specialty. It includes such categories as knowledge, psychomotor skills, managerial skills, leadership skills, technological skills, implementation, appraising of literature, screening of research proposals and mediation.

Providing external CPD activities and events is one way for the organisational perspective to shape CPD needs. However, if these external events are not well attended, then that power to shape is diminished.

Development may better be represented through the kinds of cycles to be found in a spiral as, for example, in 'Kolb's learning cycle'.[13]

Kolb states that learning involves the acquisition of abstract concepts that can be applied flexibly in a range of situations. In Kolb's learning theory, the impetus for the development of new concepts is provided by new experiences: 'Learning is the process whereby knowledge is created through the transformation of experience.'[14]

Notes

1. Greenhalgh, T. (2017) *How to Implement Evidence-Based Healthcare.* Oxford: Wiley-Blackwell.
2. See, for example, Central and North West London NHS Foundation Trust, 'Research projects, service evaluations and clinical audits.' Accessed on 5 October 2017 at www.cnwl.nhs.uk/health-professionals/icapt/research-knowledge-base/research-projects-service-evaluations-clinical-audits
3. See www.joindementiaresearch.nihr.ac.uk/content/about
4. National Institute for Health Research (2009) 'INVOLVE: Promoting public involvement in NHS, public health and social care research.' Accessed on 5 October 2017 at www.rds-london.nihr.ac.uk/RDSLondon/media/RDSContent/files/PDFs/Good-practice-in-active-public-involvement-in-research.pdf
5. The Scottish Dementia Working Group Research Sub-group, 'Core principles for involving people with dementia in research.' Accessed on 5 October 2017 at www.dementiaallianceinternational.org/wp-content/uploads/2014/08/Core-Principles_SGWG.pdf
6. Petticrew, M. and Roberts, H. (2006) *Systematic Reviews in the Social Sciences: A Practical Guide.* Malden, MA: Blackwell Publishing, p.9.
7. Sackett, D.L., Rosenberg, W.M., Muir Gray, J.A., Haynes, R.B. and Richardson, W.S. (1996) 'Evidence based medicine: What it is and what it isn't.' *BMJ 312*, 7023, 71–72, cited in Gopalakrishnan and Ganeshkumar, P. (2013) 'Systematic reviews and meta-analysis: Understanding the best evidence in primary healthcare.' *Journal of Family Medicine and Primary Care 2*, 1, 9–14.
8. Accessed on 5 October 2017 at www.dementiauk.org/for-healthcare-professionals/research-and-evaluation/geans-getting-evidence-admiral-nurse-services/
9. Alzheimer Europe, 'Ethical issues: Participating in research.' Accessed on 5 October 2017 at http://www.alzheimer-europe.org/Research/Understanding-dementia-research/Participating-in-research/Ethical-issues
10. *Collins English Dictionary*, 3rd edition (1994).

11. Redrawn from Figure 1: Steps in developing a dissemination strategy, Module 5: Disseminating the research findings, World Health Organization (2014) 'Implementation research toolkit', p.158. Accessed on 9 October 2017 at www.who.int/tdr/publications/year/2014/participant-workbook5_030414.pdf

12. www.gmc-uk.org/Item_6e___Annex_D_AoMRC_CPD_Report.pdf_28991004.pdf

13. Kolb, D.A. (1984) *Experiential Learning: Experience as the Source of Learning and Development* (Vol.1). Englewood Cliffs, NJ: Prentice-Hall.

14. Kolb 1984, p.38.

14

Leadership in transforming dementia care

According to one definition, 'leadership' is a process whereby an individual influences a group of individuals to achieve a common goal.[1]

Four types of leader, who have the responsibility of engaging the staff involved, have been identified by Damschroder and colleagues:[2]

1. **opinion leaders**, who are individuals within the organisation who have 'formal or informal influence on the attitudes and beliefs of their colleagues'

2. **formally appointed internal implementation leaders** – for example, team leaders or project leaders

3. **champions**, who dedicate themselves to supporting, marketing and overcoming resistance to change within the organisation

4. **external agents of change** who have the formal role of influencing or facilitating the process in a desirable direction.

Key drivers and policies which influence national dementia strategy and service development

BOX 14.1 NATIONAL OCCUPATIONAL STANDARDS ON CONTRIBUTING TO POLICY AND PRACTICE

National Occupational Standard SCDHSC0439 – 'Contribute to the development of organisational policy and practice' – which includes identifying potential for organisational development and presenting information and ideas to contribute to organisational development.

Arguably, a national strategy is essential for structuring care for people with dementia.

The UK National Dementia Strategy[3] stated that improved care for people with dementia can be delivered through an informed and effective dementia workforce. Subsequently, the four main 'planks' to the Prime Minister's Challenge on Dementia 2020[4] give an idea about the key drivers in current English dementia policy:

- health and care

- dementia-friendly communities

- risk reduction

- research.

It is anticipated that 'cultures of care' need to be addressed through training, improved workforce support and supervision.

Quality of care for people with dementia could be improved by enhancing nurses' leadership skills and clarifying professional values.

Evidence-based research, innovations and developments in dementia interventions and care

Our health and social care services aim to support people and their families through case detection, timely diagnosis, post-diagnostic support and adjustment, progressive and unpredictable loss of functioning, adjusting to help at home, changing lifestyle needs, hospitalisations, housing support, care home admission and complex end-of-life issues.

All of this needs to be done with respect and sensitivity to the person's lifestyle, family context and the context of the community in which they live.

If service models remain unchanged, the costs of treatment and care for people with dementia are likely to increase more rapidly than total prevalence over the same period, since care services are highly labour-intensive and wage inflation usually runs ahead of other price increases (assuming a low uptake of automatisation).

This might put considerable pressure on already stretched health and social care budgets and generate major increases in reliance on family care partners.

An excellent example of an innovation in dementia care is the MODEM project ('A comprehensive approach to MODelling outcome and costs impacts of interventions for DEMentia') which explores how changes in arrangements for the future treatment and care of people with dementia, and support for care partners, could result in better outcomes and more efficient use of resources.

The MODEM team is reviewing international evidence on effective and (potentially) cost-effective interventions in dementia care, and then using those findings, with analyses of existing and new cohort data, to model the quality-of-life and cost impacts of making these interventions more widely available in England over the period from now to 2040. The MODEM project began in 2014 and runs until February 2018. It is funded by the UK Economic and Social Research Council (ESRC) and the National Institute for Health Research (NIHR).[5]

Promoting new and evidence-based practice to challenge poor practice

---

BOX 14.2 NATIONAL OCCUPATIONAL STANDARDS ON LEADING AND MANAGING CHANGE

National Occupational Standard SCDLMCA2 – 'Lead and manage change within care services' – identifies the requirements associated with leading and managing change within care services. It includes the implementation of a shared vision for the service provision and using leadership skills to inspire those involved in the service delivery to adapt to changing needs in order to achieve positive outcomes for individuals.

Many initiatives are described in the literature that may help in the provision of better-quality care.

For example, the use of 'dementia champions' has been identified as a means of promoting best practice and ensuring that staff are supported and educated in the care of people with dementia.

A similar role is that of dementia nurse specialist (DNS), whose responsibilities include raising awareness of dementia among staff and ensuring the provision of good-quality information to people with dementia and their care partners.

The Department of Health is working with the Royal Colleges to encourage commitments to ensure that their members are capable and competent in dementia care.

Strategic clinical networks bring together those who use, provide and commission the service to make improvements in outcomes for complex patient pathways using an integrated, whole-system approach. They work in partnership with commissioners (including local government), supporting their decision-making and strategic planning.

Planning care to promote the use of appropriate, specific, evidence-based interventions

Long-term care has been defined by the World Health Organization as:

> The system of activities undertaken by informal care partners (family, friends, and/or neighbours) and/or professionals (health, social, and others) to ensure that a person who is not fully capable of self-care can maintain the highest possible quality of life, according to his or her individual preferences, with the greatest possible degree of independence, autonomy, participation, personal fulfilment, and human dignity.[6]

The functions of long-term care are generally thought to be:

- maintenance of involvement or participation in community, social and family life

- to implement environmental adaptations in housing and assistive devices

- measures to reduce disability or further deterioration through prevention or risk-reduction

- provision for identifying adequately and addressing spiritual, emotional and psychological needs

- support for family, friends and other informal care partners.

Coordination through case management is a potential alternative to improve care and to reduce costs

In a recent systematic review of the effectiveness of case management on healthcare costs and resource utilisation, case management interventions were operationalised as:

any intervention involving interaction between a case manager and patient-caregiving dyads and providing continuity and advocacy over time, support, information about community services, care and disease evolution, financial and legal advice. The case manager could also reduce fragmentation among services, monitor medication to avoid adverse reaction and give advice on behavioural management strategies tailored to the needs of patients and families. [7]

Planning for discharge could prove challenging, with delays in securing a place in residential care. These delays in transfer meant that the person with dementia might stay longer in the acute setting than was necessary and could be perceived to be 'blocking beds'.

Dawn Brooker has likened coordination to 'navigating a river'.

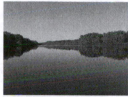

Clean and calm waters
Communities that are dementia friendly, where 'dementia' is not stigmatised, using the same facilities as everyone else, having equal rights as a citizen, having fun, having family life, schools, businesses, employers, churches, temples, synagogues, mosques

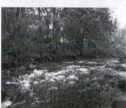

Navigating the river
Social care, providing sensitive good quality care that supports the whole family to carry on and not get overwhelmed, information, education, finances, legal, signposting, technology, adjusting, support, hugs, counselling, peer-support, getting a break, getting help at home, care homes, housing, extra care, Meeting Centres Support Programme

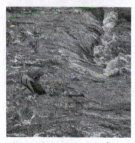

The boat hitting the rocks
Health, timely diagnosis, co-morbidities, therapeutic interventions, pharmacological and non pharmacological, specialist support in a crisis, difficult histories, specialist care in complex families, there's often more than 1 person in the boat

Figure 14.1 River analogy
Redrawn from exact text taken from a slide for a talk on 'Person Centred Leadership in Dementia Care' by Dawn Brooker for the Association for Dementia Studies, University of Worcester, UK. Reproduced by kind permission of Dawn Brooker.[8]

The need for an effective multidisciplinary approach to care and discharge planning was identified. There was also a need for mutual respect and effective communication with staff working with people with dementia in the community to facilitate the 'seamless transfer of care'.

There is a requirement for management to examine how people with dementia are introduced and moved within the acute setting. Care pathways should focus on consistency and minimal disruption wherever possible.

Care providers have long recognised the need for meaningful activity for individuals with Alzheimer's disease, and have anecdotally reported that such activity provides a sense of efficacy, reduction in depression and improved relationships with family members.

Care partners have identified physical function as an important component of quality of life for their care recipients with dementia.

The importance of demonstrating leadership in delivering compassionate person-centred care

Person-centred dementia care was first described by Kitwood,[9] who suggested the need for a new culture of care that would preserve personhood in the course of the development of the dementia disease.

Good leadership plays a key role in developing nurses' understanding of patients' needs and values, and the acceptance of new innovations to obtain successful change and a positive care culture.

By strengthening the leadership skills of nursing home leaders, it may be possible to achieve and sustain improvements that are essential to promote a better quality of life for residents.

It is suggested that care providers require appropriate support, facilitation and strong leadership if person-centred practices and compassion are to flourish.

Facilitating transformational processes within the development of person-centred care practices is considered challenging and requiring expert knowing and skills. This expertise is necessary to overcome the challenges of working within healthcare settings that always have multiple intra-relationships, sub-cultures, complexities and dynamics.

Facilitators need flexible means and a praxis approach to challenging situations that keep evolving and that do not lend themselves to straightforward technical explanations and solutions.

As person-centredness is also recognised as an enabling factor in the development of more humanistic practices, it is vital for the facilitator to know and act as a person-centred facilitator. This means to live the principles underlying person-centredness in their facilitation and to role-model person-centred relationships. 'Being' a person-centred facilitator in current dynamic healthcare contexts, however, is complex and can evoke all kind of imbalances, and has a strong historical background in the philosophy of Heidegger.[10]

High-quality, compassionate care is about people, not institutions. To maximise the effectiveness of the workforce, organisations need strong and effective leadership, and to foster a culture that encourages people to take pride in their work. Staff will need adequate training and development, and the organisation needs to support them to maintain their health and wellbeing.

Nine components (Table 14.1) have been used to conceptualise person-centred care from a review of the literature. It is noted that one key cultural characteristic of organisations that has been shown to facilitate organisational change and development is leadership style and the way that managers support and value staff. Consistent with previous studies, regular supervision was identified as an important way to support staff in providing person-centred care.

Table 14.1 Nine components to conceptualise person-centred care[11]

Respect for individuality and values	Recognises the importance of valuing people as individuals with awareness of differences, values, culture, their unique strengths, needs and rights, including the right to dignity and privacy.
Meaning	Accepts the unique perspective, reflecting the phenomenological and subjective nature of the person's experience, with self-defined goals and a potentially shared understanding of the meaning of illness.
Therapeutic alliance	Involves the possibility of genuine empathy and unconditional positive regard.
Social context and relationships	Attends to our social nature as people, with an emphasis on relationships, on our situated context of interpersonal, interconnected, mutual interdependence.
Inclusive model of health and wellbeing	Involves comfort, attachment, occupation, identity and inclusion, with attention to wellbeing and a biopsychosocial model of the person as a whole.
Expert lay knowledge	Recognises the legitimacy of the individual's or the family's expert knowledge and experience.

Shared responsibility	Suggests the sharing of power, responsibility and control, with mutual agreement on plans and reciprocity.
Communication	Encourages communication with careful, sensitive, interactional dialogue.
Autonomy	Includes the person's ability to make his or her own decisions, with independence and recognition; that individuals and families should be able to make their own choices, in accordance with principles of self-determination.
Professional as a person	Emphasises valuing staff as well as service users.

At a time when there is a desire to close the 'financial gap' in the NHS Five Year Forward View,[12] yet demand upon and public expectations of the health system are rising, it is vital that organisations look at how they use their available resources and workforce, and consider how things can be done more efficiently.

The importance of quality assurance and service improvement

The terms 'quality' and 'quality improvement' mean different things to different people in different circumstances. This can be confusing.

Within healthcare, there is no universally accepted definition of 'quality'. However, the following definition, from the US Institute of Medicine, is often used (cited in Beaulieu[13]): quality is 'the degree to which health services for individuals and populations increase the likelihood of desired health outcomes and are consistent with current professional knowledge'.

The Institute of Medicine has identified six dimensions of healthcare quality.[14] These state that healthcare must be:

- safe

- timely

- effective

- efficient

- person-centred

- equitable.

There is no single definition of quality improvement. However, a number of definitions describe it as a systematic approach that uses specific techniques to improve quality. One important ingredient in successful and sustained improvement is the way in which the change is introduced and implemented. Taking a consistent approach is key.

Training and supporting team members to meet the needs of people with dementia

BOX 14.3 NATIONAL OCCUPATIONAL STANDARDS ON CHANGE AND LEADERSHIP

National Occupational Standard CFAM&LBA2 – 'Provide leadership in your area of responsibility' – is about providing direction to people in a defined area or part of an organisation and motivating and supporting them to achieve the vision and objectives for the area.

National Occupational Standard CFAM&LCA3 – 'Engage people in change' – is about engaging people – both those within your organisation and other stakeholders who are affected – in change processes.

Nowhere is leadership more crucial to improving care quality than on the front line – in wards, clinics and general practices.

Leadership at the front line is often best performed by clinicians (including doctors, nurses, social workers and Allied Health Professionals), together with general managers.

Practitioners and professionals are well placed to take charge of the factors known to affect outcomes – teamwork, inter-professional communication, standardised care processes and process compliance – not least because of the credibility they have with colleagues providing care directly.

One of the challenges facing leaders is to identify goals that can unify and engage a team with diverse professional backgrounds while reflecting the organisation's values and priorities.

Developing goals from the bottom up can conflict with the tendency to set goals centrally. Goals must be specific, challenging, measurable and realistic.

Improving how the team works with other teams – inside and beyond the organisation – should always be a key goal.

Crucially, leaders must give teams feedback based on reliable data about their performance so that they can improve their effectiveness. Making good progress towards the goal should be celebrated.

The importance of collaborative working in the provision of support, care and services for people with dementia, their families and care partners

Reaching shared decision-making in the context of dementia is even more difficult because people with dementia experience increasing difficulties in making decisions due to cognitive decline.

They want to be involved in decisions about their lives as long as possible, but realise that over time they will increasingly have to rely on their informal care partners. In addition, informal care partners experience difficulties in deciding for their loved ones.

Collaboration encompasses multiple participants working together to move towards a certain course of action. Rather than focusing on reaching consensus, collaboration emphasises the process of working together in reaching decisions.

The roles and responsibilities of different agencies involved in dementia care

BOX 14.4 NATIONAL OCCUPATIONAL STANDARDS ON COLLABORATIVE WORKING

National Occupational Standard SCDHSC0433 – 'Develop joint working arrangements for health and social care services' – outlines the requirements when you develop joint working agreements and practices to deliver health and social care services in the most effective ways.

National Occupational Standard SFHGEN126 – 'Monitor, evaluate and improve inter-agency services for addressing health and wellbeing needs' – covers monitoring, evaluating and leading teams to improve delivering inter-agency services for addressing health and wellbeing needs. It covers working with both service users and providers.

Perhaps the most important common guiding principle for all multidisciplinary/integrated teams, regardless of organisational setting, is having a shared commitment to the delivery of person-centred coordinated care from the perspective of the individual: 'I can plan my care with people who work together to understand me and my care partner(s), allow me control, and bring together services to achieve the outcomes important to me.'

Many reports and publications have been considered in an attempt to identify and draw out the common principles/key traits to successful multidisciplinary team working which could collectively be summarised around leadership, relationships, culture, clinical engagement, developing the workforce, information (data and intelligence), communication, and commissioning – more recently, co-commissioning and outcomes-based commissioning.

NHS England supports the use of 'multiagency working'. Multiagency working is important for challenging principles:

- cultural boundaries across pathways – whether professional or sectorial

- system and bureaucratic boundaries to access joined-up specialised and non-specialised services and equipment provision

- funding and budgets.[15]

Multiagency working is important for creating opportunities:

- Transferable flexible guidelines, tools, techniques allowing the benefits of knowledge, skills and expertise to be shared and accessible across pathways – whether health, social care or public health for the benefit of all.

- Focus on health, health outcomes and supporting the client or patient to maintain or improve their own health.

- Encourages leadership within a culture of collaboration, working with and across boundaries and along pathways based upon the need(s) of the patients.[16]

The principles of equality and diversity for access to and delivery of services

The cornerstone of the Equality Act 2010[17] is the statutory public-sector equality duty, which requires all public bodies and those performing public functions to eliminate unlawful discrimination against groups of people with defined protected characteristics, advance equality of opportunity and mitigate against threatening behaviour.

Gender equality in access to and delivery of services is of huge concern. Around the world, more women than men live with dementia. As a known risk factor for dementia, the global aging population will contribute to a rapid increase of dementia, particularly for women. To develop dementia plans and strategies that will work for women at every stage of their life, national policy makers and civil society advocates can utilise a range of international policy frameworks including the World Health Organization's draft 'Global action plan on the public health response to dementia 2017–2025'.[18]

These frameworks give clear guidance – and in some cases obligations – as to how national dementia responses can take on a gendered perspective.

The absence of gender perspectives in current dementia policy and programming points to the vital significance of women-focused non-governmental organisations collaborating with dementia specialists and government policy makers to mainstream gender equality into future responses.

Mechanisms need to be in place to monitor these frameworks to ensure implementation to protect the rights and needs of people living with dementia and to identify the most suitable methods to drive women higher up the 'dementia agenda'.

Notes

1. Northouse, P.G. (2013) *Leadership Theory and Practice* (6th edition). Thousand Oaks, CA: SAGE.
2. Damschroder L.J., Aron, D.C., Keith, R.E., Kirsh, S.R., Alexander J.A. and Lowery J.C. (2009) 'Fostering implementation of health services research findings into practice: A consolidated framework for advancing implementation science.' *Implementation Science 4*, 50.
3. Department of Health (2009) 'Living Well with Dementia: A national dementia strategy.' Accessed on 5 October 2017 at www.gov.uk/government/publications/living-well-with-dementia-a-national-dementia-strategy
4. Department of Health (2015) 'Prime Minister's Challenge on Dementia 2020.' Accessed on 5 October 2017 at www.gov.uk/government/uploads/system/uploads/attachment_data/file/414344/pm-dementia2020.pdf
5. See Comas-Herrera, A., Knapp, M., Wittenberg, R., Banerjee ,S. *et al.* MODEM Project Group (2017) 'MODEM: A comprehensive approach to modelling outcome and costs impacts of interventions for dementia. Protocol paper.' BMC Health Services Research 17, 25. Accessed on 5 October 2017 at http://eprint.ncl.ac.uk/file_store/production/232504/B1969A36-C9D1-40C5-9307-63C6E76F00B9.pdf
6. www.euro.who.int/en/health-topics/Life-stages/healthy-ageing/data-and-statistics/health-and-social-care-systems

7. Pimouguet, C., Lavaud, T., Dartigues, J.F. and Helmer, C. (2010) 'Dementia case management effectiveness on health care costs and resource utilization: A systematic review of randomized controlled trials.' *Journal of Nutrition, Health and Aging 14*, 8, 669–676.

8. See www.ksseducation.hee.nhs.uk/files/2014/08/Person-Centred-Leadership-in-Dementia-Care-Professor-Dawn-Brooker.pdf

9. Kitwood, T. (1997) *Dementia Reconsidered: The Person Comes First.* Buckingham: Open University Press.

10. Stanford Encyclopedia of Philosophy, Martin Heidegger (1889–1976). Accessed on 5 October 2017 at https://plato.stanford.edu/entries/heidegger

11. Adapted from Box 1 (Framework of components of person-centred care), Kirkley, C., Bamford, C., Poole, M., Arksey, H., Hughes, J. and Bond, J. (2011) 'The impact of organisational culture on the delivery of person-centred care in services providing respite care and short breaks for people with dementia.' *Health and Social Care in the Community 19*, 4, 438–448. doi: 10.1111/j.1365-2524.2011.00998.x

12. NHS England (2014) 'Five Year Forward View.' Accessed on 5 October at www.england.nhs.uk/wp-content/uploads/2014/10/5yfv-web.pdf

13. Cited in Beaulieu, M.-D. (2013) 'Assessing quality: Giving patients a voice.' *Canadian Family Physician 59*, 3, 317. Accessed on 5 October 2017 at www.ncbi.nlm.nih.gov/pmc/articles/PMC3596213

14. The Health Foundation (2013) 'Quality improvement made simple: What everyone should know about health care quality improvement.' Accessed on 5 October 2017 at www.health.org.uk/sites/health/files/QualityImprovementMadeSimple.pdf

15. NHS England (2014) 'MDT Development: Working toward an effective multidisciplinary/multiagency team.' Accessed on 5 October 2017 at www.england.nhs.uk/wp-content/uploads/2015/01/mdt-dev-guid-flat-fin.pdf

16. NHS England (2014) 'MDT Development: Working toward an effective multidisciplinary/multiagency team.' Accessed on 5 October 2017 at www.england.nhs.uk/wp-content/uploads/2015/01/mdt-dev-guid-flat-fin.pdf

17. See www.legislation.gov.uk/ukpga/2010/15/contents?

18. Accessed on 5 October 2017 at www.who.int/mental_health/neurology/dementia/zero_draft_dementia_action_plan_5_09_16.pdf

Afterword

This 'afterword' picks up many of the themes in Chapter 13 ('Research and evidence-based practice in dementia care') of this book.

The structure for this book was provided by the Department of Health which commissioned the 'Dementia Core Skills Education and Training Framework'.[1] This was developed by Health Education England and Skills for Health.

The Dementia Core Skills Education and Training Framework provides a detailed specification of minimum learning outcomes at tiers 1, 2 and 3 for the health and care workforce.

To draw maximum benefit from this, you are strongly advised to read widely around dementia anyway.

Examples of important and up-to-date references include the following.

- *The British National Formulary* is a United Kingdom pharmaceutical reference book that contains a wide spectrum of information and advice on prescribing and pharmacology, along with specific facts and details about all medicines that are made available within the UK National Health Service. It is available online (www.bnf.org/products/bnf-online).

- The National Institute for Health and Clinical Excellence (NICE) publishes authoritative guidance and guidelines to support the very best evidence-based care of people with dementia cared for within health and social services. Everything is available online and easy to access (www.nice.org.uk).

- The Social Care Institute for Excellence (SCIE) is an improvement support agency and an independent charity working with adults', families' and children's care and support services across the UK. They publish much of interest to the general public and professionals alike online (www.scie.org.uk).

• The National Occupational Standards (NOS) are statements of the standards of performance for individuals when carrying out functions in the workplace, together with specification of the underpinning knowledge and understanding. The standards are all easily available online (www.ukstandards.org.uk).

Identifying a gap to study

It is worth looking at the National Institute for Health Research (NIHR) website: www.nihr.ac.uk

The people who carry out research are mostly the same doctors and healthcare professionals who treat people across the NHS. Their aim is to find better ways of looking after patients and keeping people healthy.

There are many different types of research, covering a range of activities, from working in a scientific laboratory to carefully noting patterns of health and disease to developing new treatments.

Healthcare professionals are being encouraged to base their clinical practice on research-based knowledge. Every year, hundreds of professional journals are published, containing thousands of reports of research studies. The healthcare professional searching the literature is likely to discover a number of sources which will vary in terms of quality, comprehensibility and relevance to practice.

A research project begins with an idea which is then transformed into a research question. Many questions for research that can lead to patient benefit arise from observations made by health professionals in the NHS and social care.

A research question is a clear, focused and concise statement that conveys the objectives of the research and its potential findings. It determines the success of a research process and should drive the development of a research protocol. A research question should be expressed in simple, straightforward language.

Doctors and healthcare professionals know a great deal about health, disease and treatments, but there are still some things that are unknown. Research can help find answers, filling gaps in knowledge and changing the way that doctors and healthcare professionals deliver care.

It is worth looking at the Cochrane Dementia and Cognitive Improvement Group (http://dementia.cochrane.org), based at Oxford University in the Radcliffe Department of Medicine. Excellent blogs of interest can be found on www.evidentlycochrane.net. Their remit includes both global cognitive impairment and focal cognitive impairments occurring in the context of brain disease, but many of their reviews are indeed concerned specifically with dementia.

Reading a paper

The practical question to ask, then, about a new piece of research is not 'Has anyone ever done a similar study?' but 'Does this new research add to the literature in any way?' Ask 'Who is the study about, and who is this study aimed at?'

Before assuming that the results of a paper are applicable to your own practice, ask yourself the following questions:

- Who was included in the study and why?

- Were the subjects studied in 'real-life' circumstances?

- Was the design of the study sensible?

  You should always look for evidence in the paper that the outcome measure has been objectively validated. Was systematic bias avoided or minimised? Systematic bias is defined as anything that erroneously influences the conclusions about groups and distorts comparisons. Think about how different study designs call for different steps to reduce systematic bias.

- Was assessment 'blind'? (A blind – or blinded – experiment is an experiment in which information about the test is kept from the participant, to reduce or eliminate bias, until after a trial outcome is known. It is understood that bias may be intentional or unconscious. If both tester and subject are blinded, the trial is called a double-blind experiment.)

  Even the most rigorous attempt to achieve a comparable control group will be wasted effort if the people who assess the outcome know which group the patient they are assessing was allocated to.

- Were preliminary statistical questions dealt with?

  Three important numbers can often be found in the methods section of a paper: the size of the sample; the duration of follow-up; and the completeness of follow-up.

- Are these results credible?

BOX A.1 OVERVIEW OF COMMON TYPES OF STUDY DESIGN

Randomised controlled trials

In a randomised controlled trial, systematic bias is (in theory) avoided by selecting a sample of participants from a particular population and allocating them randomly to the different groups.

Non-randomised ('other') controlled clinical trials

As a general rule, if the paper you are looking at is a non-randomised controlled clinical trial, you must use your common sense to decide if the baseline differences between the intervention and control groups are likely to have been so great as to invalidate any differences attributed to the effects of the intervention.

Cohort studies

In a cohort study, two (or more) groups of people are selected on the basis of differences in their exposure to a particular agent, and followed up to see how many in each group develop a particular disease, complication or other outcome.

Case-control studies

Case-control studies are where the experiences of individuals with and without a particular disease are analysed retrospectively to identify putative causative events.

Reflective learning

Reflective learning is a way of allowing students to step back from their learning experience to help them develop critical thinking skills and improve on future performance by analysing their experience.

Lioba Howatson-Jones (2016) provides:[2]

Reflection has been defined variously as accessing previous experience helping to develop tacit and intuitive knowledge, a transformative process that changes individuals and their actions, and a way to reach awareness of how and why things have occurred. 'Tacit knowledge' is about having a common understanding about something and 'intuitive' means sensitive to links with previous experience.

Understanding assessment criteria and acting on feedback is also a way of encouraging students to reflect on what they have learned and how they will improve.

A simple way of getting to grips with the idea of reflection is to set ten minutes aside each week to write a 'learning log'. A learning log is a bit like a diary or portfolio, but it has set headings that encourage you to record important details.

Here are four things to record in a simple learning log:

- the experience/situation/event

- your initial reactions to it

- what you did

- what you learned from the experience/situation/event.

The reader is strongly encouraged to refer to How to *Read a Paper: The Basics of Evidence-Based Medicine* (Fifth edition) by Trisha Greenhalgh (Wiley Blackwell/BMJ Books).

Most of all, good luck!

Notes

1. See www.skillsforhealth.org.uk/services/item/176-dementia-core-skills-education-and-training-framework
2. Howatson-Jones, L. (2016) *Reflective Practice in Nursing*, 3rd edition, London: Sage Publications, p.7.

Bibliography

The main reference is, of course, the Dementia Core Skills Education and Training Framework.

The Dementia Core Skills Education and Training Framework was commissioned and funded by the Department of Health and developed in collaboration by Skills for Health and Health Education England (HEE) in partnership with Skills for Care. Development of the framework was guided by an Expert Group including a wide range of health and social care organisations, relevant Royal Colleges and education providers. www.skillsforhealth.org.uk/services/itcm/176-dementia-core-skills-education-and-training-framework

Other useful publications include the following:

Brooker, D. and Latham, I. (2016) *Person-Centred Dementia Care*, 2nd edition. London: Jessica Kingsley Publishers.

Dementia UK, Higher Education for Dementia Network (HEDN) (2013) 'Curriculum for UK Dementia Education.' Accessed on 5 October 2017 at https://www.dementiauk.org/for-healthcare-professionals/free-resources/download-the-curriculum-for-demenita-education

Department of Health (2015) 'Prime Minister's Challenge on Dementia 2020.' www.gov.uk/government/publications/prime-ministers-challenge-on-dementia-2020

Hodges, J.R. (2007) *Cognitive Assessment for Clinicians*. Oxford: Oxford University Press.

Husain, M. and Schott, J. (2016) *Oxford Textbook of Cognitive Neurology and Dementia* (Oxford Textbooks in Clinical Neurology). Oxford: Oxford University Press.

London Dementia Strategic Clinical Network (2014) 'Guide to Dementia Training for Health and Social Care Staff in London: Improving Quality of Care.' Accessed on 5 October 2017 at https:// hee.nhs.uk/sites/default/files/documents/Guide%20to%20 Dementia%20Training%20for%20Health%20and%20Social%20 Care%20Staff%20in%20London.pdf

McCormack, B. and McCance, T. (eds) (2017) *Person-Centred Practice in Nursing and Health Care*, 2nd edition. Oxford: Wiley-Blackwell.

Rahman, S. (2015) *Living Better with Dementia: Good Practice and Innovation for the Future.* London: Jessica Kingsley Publishers. *This book includes a description of the drive to reduce inappropriate prescribing of antipsychotics, and reviews many aspects, including stigma and delirium.*

Rahman, S. (2017) *Enhancing Health and Wellbeing in Dementia: A Person-Centred Integrated Care Approach.* London: Jessica Kingsley Publishers. *This book gives an account of a 'living well' pathway, comparable to the NHS England Transformation Network.*

Worcestershire Health and Care NHS Trust (2011) *Stand by Me: Promoting Good Communication with People Living with Dementia and Their Families.* Accessed on 5 October 2017 at www.worcester.ac.uk/ documents/Stand_By_Me_Book_sample.pdf